HOW TO LOSE
WEIGHT

A Veteran's 200-Pound Natural
Weight Loss in One Year

CRISTIAN LOPEZ

Interior Layout by: Saqib Arshad

DISCLAIMER

This book shares the author's personal experiences and opinions. It is provided for educational and motivational purposes only and is not medical, nutritional, or mental-health advice. It is not a substitute for professional diagnosis, treatment, or individualized guidance. Always consult a qualified healthcare professional, especially if you have medical conditions, use a CPAP, take medications, or are considering fasting or a new exercise program.

Use of the information herein is at your own risk. The author and publisher disclaim all liability for any injury, loss, or damages resulting from the use or misuse of this material. Results vary with genetics, health status, effort, and adherence. If you experience dizziness, chest pain, shortness of breath, or other concerning symptoms, stop immediately and seek medical care.

EXTENDED DISCLAIMER & READER NOTICE

The strategies described in this book reflect the author's personal journey and are presented for informational purposes only. They are not intended as a substitute for medical, nutritional, psychological, or other professional advice, diagnosis, or treatment. Do not disregard, delay, or modify professional guidance because of something you have read here.

Always consult your physician or another qualified provider before beginning any new nutrition approach, fasting protocol, supplement, cardio or strength routine, or sleep/CPAP adjustments—particularly if you have chronic conditions (including but not limited to diabetes, cardiovascular disease, or sleep apnea), take prescription medications, are pregnant or nursing, or have a history of disordered eating.

Exercise and dietary changes involve inherent risks. Stop immediately and seek medical attention if you experience faintness, chest pain, unusual shortness of breath, or other concerning symptoms. The author and publisher make no guarantees of specific outcomes; results vary depending on individual factors and adherence. To the fullest extent permitted by law, they disclaim liability for any loss, injury, or damages arising from the use or misuse of this content.

Brand names and trademarks remain the property of their respective owners and are used for identification only. Any testimonials or examples included are illustrative and not typical; they do not guarantee similar results.

ACKNOWLEDGEMENTS

To my fellow veterans and to anyone carrying invisible battles, traction starts here. Discipline stacked daily can win the fight for your health, your life, your freedom.

DEDICATION

*To everyone ready to take their life back,
this book is your blueprint.*

TABLE OF CONTENTS

Introduction: The Traction Blueprint   1

Chapter 1:   You'll Never Change   3

Chapter 2:   Traction > Motivation   7

Chapter 3:   The War Plan: First 30 Days   15

Chapter 4:   Protein or Nothing   21

Chapter 5:   Grams Don't Lie   25

Chapter 6:   MTKU: Move to Kill the Urge   29

Chapter 7:   Steps = Sanity   35

Chapter 8:   Sleep Debt = Snack Debt   41

Chapter 9:   Starve The Traps   45

Chapter 10:   Travel, Parties, Pressure: Still in Control   49

Chapter 11:   Proof Over Plateaus   57

Chapter 12:   Lose Loose Skin   61

Chapter 13:   Protein vs. "Protein"   73

Chapter 14:   Hungers Psychology   79

Chapter 15:   Chakra Energy   87

Chapter 16:   The Days We Don't Want to Show Up   107

Chapter 17:   Environment Is Everything   115

Chapter 18:   This Is Not a Diet   131

Chapter 19:   The New You Is Non-Negotiable   137

Chapter 20:   Survival to Significance   143

Chapter 21:   The Prospect of War   151

Chapter 22:   The Recovery Key   157

Connect with the Author   177

The Traction Blueprint

This isn't a diet book. It's a blueprint for traction. It's the system that rewired my body and can rewire yours. I didn't lose 200 pounds because I found the perfect program, got lucky, or stayed motivated. Motivation fades. Luck never shows up. I lost the weight because I stopped negotiating with weakness and started stacking proof. The same discipline that builds millionaires in business builds transformations in the body. The principle is identical: *Traction beats motivation. Proof beats promises. Systems beat shortcuts.* Mindset matters, but mindset without mechanics fails. Results come from a few non-negotiables executed with ruthless consistency:

▶ Protein or Nothing. Anchor every day in nutrition that fuels change.
▶ Grams Don't Lie. Weigh it, track it, own it.
▶ MTKU (Move To Kill the Urge). Cravings don't get a meeting. They get movement.
▶ Steps = Sanity. Mileage is medicine.
▶ Sleep Debt = Snack Debt. Win the night, win the kitchen.
▶ Starve the Traps. Engineer your environment so relapse can't find oxygen.

I've lived this system. At my lowest, I was 387 pounds and I couldn't recognize the man staring back at me in the mirror. I felt trapped in a body that didn't match who I knew I could be, ashamed to be seen in public, and tired of breaking promises to myself.

So, I started small. One silent driveway lap at a time. Proof stacked slowly, then relentlessly, until the lies in my head had nowhere left to stand.

That same blueprint that rebuilt me has since helped others do the same for breaking cycles of failure, restoring health, and finally ending the pattern of starting over.

This book is not theory. It's the exact *Traction Blueprint* system that rewires bodies and lives. No shortcuts. No gimmicks. Just the non-negotiables that build proof, stack momentum, and make relapse nearly impossible.

- ▶ The War Plan. A 30 day system to ignite momentum.
- ▶ Food Rules. Simple, repeatable, non-negotiable.
- ▶ Crisis Protocols. What to do when you plateau or relapse.
- ▶ Identity Lock In. The system that makes the new you permanent.

If you're tired of quitting, tired of chasing sparks that fade, and tired of carrying shame that never leaves. Then turn the page.

This is the system that doesn't care how you feel. It only cares what you do.

CLS: The Cristian Lopez System.

Change. Lose. Stack.

Change your identity. Lose the weight. Stack proof forever.

CHAPTER 1

You'll Never Change

All my life, I heard the same words: *Your fat. You're lazy. You'll never change.*

They weren't just insults from other people. They became my own voice, whispering in my head, poisoning me day after day.

By 2021, I was nearly 400 pounds. My man boobs rolled into my overhanging belly, love handles spilling over my waist. But somehow, I didn't see it. I told myself the same lie every day: *I'm just getting through it. Tomorrow I'll change.* But tomorrow never came.

We had just moved to a small town called Lake City, Florida. I thought it would be a place to set roots. Instead, it was a gateway town for drugs, cults, and broken systems. Unfortunately, we bought the house sight unseen. My plan was the same as always. Make it work. Survive, don't act.

Then came the doctor's visit.

The nurse had me step on the scale. "Dang, you're that big," he muttered. The number lit up like a death sentence: *387.* Shame flooded me. I felt like I needed to apologize just for existing.

The nurse walked me to another room. There sat the doctor, hunched over his computer, typing and reading in silence. He didn't look at me. He just studied the screen, his fingers clicking the keys like he already knew my death sentence.

Then, without a word, he began unbuttoning his shirt. One button. Then another. Until his chest was bare. Gray hair across his skin, and a scar running straight down the middle like a warning sign.

He leaned closer, the scar only a soda can away from my face.

He pointed at it.
"I was obese too," he said. "I almost died from it. This scar is from my open-heart surgery."

Then he leaned forward, eyes locked on mine.
"You have the most severe case of sleep apnea I've ever seen. Your blood pressure is dangerously high. You're pre diabetic. If you don't change, you won't live another year."

That should have wrecked me. But instead, I walked out of that office, stopped at a drive thru, and ordered a milkshake on the way home. That's where I was, killing myself one sip at a time.

The Lie We All Hear

My words were *"You'll never change."*
Maybe yours sound different:

- *"You'll always be big."*
- *"You never stick to anything."*
- *"It's just genetics. This is who you are."*

Different words. Same poison.

When I got home that day, everything changed.
My daughter, barely walking and talking, came running up to me. "Dada! Dada!" she said, with that innocent joy only a child can have.

And in that moment, it hit me like a freight train: if I didn't fight for my life, she'd grow up without a father. I knew damn well what that meant. A girl without her father is left vulnerable to a world that doesn't care if she survives it.

I wasn't leaving my daughter fatherless. Not here. Not like this.

That day, my life stopped being about survival. It became about war.

The Weapon That Wins

Motivation didn't save me. Hope didn't save me. *Proof did.*

One driveway lap. One skipped snack. One pound lost.
That's how you kill the lie. Not with hype. With evidence.

Proof stacks higher than doubt.
And once you stack enough proof, the voice that says *"You'll never change"* goes silent.

Your First Dare

Now it's your turn.
Write down the lie that's been running your life. Don't dress it up. Don't soften it. Write it raw.

Then today, stack one piece of proof against it. Walk. Weigh. Log your food. Skip the snack. Just one.

You don't need to feel ready. You need to stack proof.

The Next Wire

That was the first wire I had to rewire in my life, the wire that started everything.

But killing a lie isn't enough. To lose the weight for good, you have to become someone new.

That's what comes next: *Identity.*
Because if you only lose pounds, you'll gain them back. But if you become a new person, the weight can't come back.

CHAPTER 2

Traction > Motivation

What does motivation look like to you?

It may show up in different forms, but it acts the same for everyone. Motivation will get the engine started, but it's not the fuel that keeps it running.

Hype fades. Proof stacks.

There were issues I had to attack if I was going to survive this journey. The first was food.

I created eating windows, clear times when I could eat and times when I couldn't. No in-between. This is what you call a fasted state. A fast is simply the time between your last meal and your next.

Note: *That's where the word "breakfast" comes from: you break the fast.*

My fasts lasted a minimum of 14 hours daily.

Tip: Use your sleeping hours as part of your fast.

There are many ways to fast, but the key is keeping your body in fat-burning mode. After about 12 hours without food, your body starts tapping into fat stores for energy. The longer you hold the line, the more disciplined your body becomes.

The First Miles

The morning after my declaration of war, I woke up and dragged myself to the elliptical. Fifteen minutes, fasted. That was all I could handle. My legs burned. My lungs screamed. But I did it.

For the first week, I stuck with it. Every morning, fasted cardio. At first it was 15 minutes, then 20, then 30. By day seven, I pushed myself to two hours.

Two hours. Me, the guy who couldn't even walk without wheezing.

I realized something: *proof stacks higher than doubt.*

And I refused to let doubt bury my proof.

Cold Turkey

The cravings hit hard. The old voices tried to drag me back. Just one soda. Just one binge. Skip today's workout, you've done enough.

The motivation ran out.
Discipline was the only thing that could keep my story alive.

I refused to give weakness a vote. Every time a negative thought showed up, I attacked it with movement. I marched harder, pushed faster, punished the weakness. I trained my body to obey my mind.

And then I found out my wife was pregnant. Suddenly, it wasn't just one child I was fighting for. It was two.

So I went cold turkey:

- No fast food.
- No soda.
- Strict portions.
- Every gram of food weighed.
- CPAP nightly.
- Daily fast.

Chicken, rice, nonfat Greek yogurt, spinach, fruit. Kitchen closed by 7 p.m. Bed by 9 p.m. CPAP strapped on. Discipline became my lifeline.

Weakness doesn't get a vote. Because integrity with yourself is the only vote that counts.

STOP waiting until tomorrow.
STOP telling yourself you'll start after the holidays.
STOP making promises and start stacking proof.

There's no perfect timing where the stars align. The perfect timing is now.

Mailbox to Mailbox

Self-assessments are crucial for growth. I'm talking about a hard, honest look in the mirror. *No excuses, no sugar-coating.*

Once I accomplished two hours on the elliptical, I knew it was time to change. I didn't stick to the machine just to master it. The goal wasn't ego, it was growth. Growth meant challenging myself daily, showing up at 100%, adapting to every obstacle, and attacking problems head-on instead of going around them.

Life gives you a million reasons not to show up. You only need one reason why you must.

At first, I was too ashamed to be seen even walking in my neighborhood. I couldn't remember the last time I ran.

When's the last time you sprinted full speed?

My first cardio sessions outside were laps in my own driveway. Just me, the Florida air, and the sound of my footsteps. Back and forth until I hit five miles.

It was brutal. My whole lower body screamed. The elliptical hadn't prepared me for this. More than once, I puked in the Florida heat. To adjust, I started heat training, 2.5 miles in the daytime, 2.5 miles at night.

Tip: *Invest in good quality shoes.*

Eventually, I built the endurance and confidence to walk five miles daily around my neighborhood.

My fasting window reset my body to burn fat instead of sugar. It wasn't magic, it was math. Less time eating = fewer chances to binge.

I locked in on my numbers:

- ▶ 200 grams of protein.
- ▶ 90 grams of carbs.
- ▶ Less than 1,000 mg sodium.
- ▶ Always in a calorie deficit.

My goal weight was 180 pounds, so I followed a soldier's formula: 1–2 grams of protein per pound of goal body weight.

Tip: Base your numbers on your goal weight. Calorie deficit = weight loss.

Every step, every day, felt like hell. But I realized something: cardio and fatigue are illusions. They're just stories your body tells to make you quit.

Quick Note: When your body says it's done, you've only reached about 30% of your potential. That means 70% is still on the table.

So I snapped back into military cadence. I remembered the freezing Chicago winters, marching through the snow. Knees high. Hoo-rah! Sweat pouring in the cold, step after step.

At first, I couldn't make it a mile. So I made checkpoints: mailbox to mailbox. Run past one, walk two. Run past one, walk two. Then one-for-one. Eventually, I ran them all.

Fatigue is an illusion. Quitting is real.

Sacred Miles

I didn't have fancy equipment or a trainer. I made do with what I had. And I learned the truth: cardio isn't about talent or performance. It's about not quitting.

That expensive watch won't make you run faster.

So I surrendered fully to the pain. I stopped expecting it to be easy. I expected to suffer. That surrender became my power.

When I wanted to quit, I pictured the version of me I hated

The man too depressed to leave the house.

The husband whose wife would eventually leave.

The father whose kids wouldn't want anything to do with him.

The man in the mirror I couldn't recognize.

That *fear became my fuel.*

The adrenaline carried me through. I shattered doubt with discipline. If I was sleeping, hitting my miles, eating in a deficit, and staying consistent, the results would come. Brick by brick. Empire by empire.

By three months, I had lost **110 pounds. Over 450 miles** completed.

None of those miles mattered by themselves. But together, they changed everything.

No story is worth telling without setbacks. No goal is worth setting if you don't question whether you can actually reach it. That's the beauty, humans are built to break limits. That's how you become limitless.

As long as it takes. In it to win it.

Every mile was proof. Every drop of sweat was validation. *Confidence doesn't come from watching other; it comes from doing what's right, even when you're alone.*

I ran those miles alone. No crowd. No cheerleaders. No training partners. Just me.

But that didn't make it meaningless.

It made it sacred.

Discipline is the only hype that lasts.

The Wire You Never Cut

Did you know foxes live in dens with only their closest family? That's their foxhole.

So who's in your foxhole?

My wife. My daughter. My newborn on the way. They became my red wires, the wires you never cut, the ones you protect at all costs.

That's why motivation didn't save me. Motivation would've quit on day three.

You must find your why, and make it unbreakable. Make it your red wire.

Motivation can spark traction, but it won't fuel the journey.

Traction saved me.

Step after step. Brick after brick. Mile after mile.

Motivation got me started. Traction kept me moving. That's why *discipline > motivation.*

Your Turn

Ready or not? Doesn't matter!

Now it's your turn.

Don't wait to feel ready. Don't wait for perfect conditions.

Pick one thing today. Just one. Do it again tomorrow. Then the next day.

Hack: To kill procrastination, just go.

Stack your proof until your excuses choke on it.

Because once traction takes hold, motivation isn't even necessary. It becomes habit.

The proof becomes your fuel.

Motivation fades. Traction builds.

Start small. Stay ruthless. Stack proof.

CHAPTER 3

The War Plan: First 30 Days

This isn't a diet. This isn't a workout program.

This is war.

The enemy is weakness. The battlefield is your daily life.

And this **30 day** war plan is your first campaign.

If you execute it without compromise, you will win. It doesn't matter if you're 400 pounds or already fit. The rules of war don't change.

Fail to plan, plan to fail.

Phase 1: Days 1–10 – Discipline First

The first 10 days are not about perfection. They're about proving to yourself that weakness doesn't get a vote anymore. You are setting the rules of engagement.

Daily Non-Negotiables:

▶ **Fasting Window:** Minimum 14 hours. Use your sleeping hours to cover most of it. Example: Eat between 10 a.m. and 8 p.m. only.

Why: After about 12 hours without food, your body starts shifting from burning sugar (glucose) to burning fat for energy. Fasting resets your hunger hormones and teaches your body discipline.

Food

- ▸ Protein first. Minimum: 150–200g daily (adjust by goal weight).
- ▸ Eliminate soda, fast food, fried foods, added sugar.
- ▸ Keep carbs under 100g. Choose rice, oats, fruit, or vegetables, **nothing processed.**
- ▸ Sodium under 1,000mg.

Why: Protein preserves muscle while you lose fat. Carbs fuel performance but too many keep you from burning fat. High sodium bloats your body and raises blood pressure.

Hydration: Minimum 1 gallon of water.

Why: Most cravings are actually dehydration. Water controls appetite and keeps performance high.

Sleep: Bedtime set. 7–8 hours, CPAP if needed.

Why: Sleep regulates testosterone, growth hormone, and recovery. Lack of it kills fat loss.

Movement: 30 minutes of fasted cardio daily (walk, elliptical, march). Doesn't matter how slow. It matters that you move.

Why: Fasted cardio accelerates fat use and teaches your body to burn fuel efficiently.

Mantras for Phase 1:

- ▸ *Weakness doesn't get a vote.*
- ▸ *Start small. Stay ruthless.*
- ▸ *Discipline is the only hype that lasts.*

By Day 10, you're not chasing results. You're building a streak. Every day you complete the list, you prove you're in control.

Phase 2: Days 11–20 – Endurance

Now the body fights back. Cravings scream. Excuses multiply. Fatigue sets in. This is where most people quit.

But you're not most people.

Your mission is endurance.

Daily Non-Negotiables (Build on Phase 1):

Fasting: Extend to 16 hours minimum. Example: 12 p.m. – 8 p.m. eating window.

Why: Longer fasting improves insulin sensitivity and teaches your body to use stored fat more efficiently.

Food: Protein 200g daily (based on goal weight). Carbs locked at 75–90g.

Why: Higher protein keeps you full and protects muscle. Keeping carbs moderate ensures fat continues to drop without killing performance.

Movement: 45–60 minutes of cardio. Split into two sessions if needed (example: 2.5 miles AM, 2.5 miles PM).

Why: Splitting cardio builds endurance and calorie burn while keeping recovery manageable.

Strength: Add 2 sessions per week. Push-ups, squats, pull-ups, or gym lifts. Doesn't matter how many reps — it matters you start stacking strength.

Why: Muscle burns calories even at rest. Strength training ensures your weight loss is fat loss, not muscle loss.

Mindset Drill: Write down one excuse that came up today. Burn it on paper. Excuses don't survive the battlefield.

Mantras for Phase 2:

> ▸ *Fatigue is an illusion. Quitting is real.*
> ▸ *Life gives you a million reasons not to show up. You only need one reason why you must.*

By Day 20, your body will change. Clothes fit differently. Energy spikes midday. Cravings lose their grip. But the biggest change is internal, proof is stacking.

Phase 3: Days 21–30 – Proof Stacks

The final 10 days are about consolidation. You've already proven you can do it. Now you weaponize consistency.

Daily Non-Negotiables (Refine & Harden):

Fasting: 16–18 hours. Your body adapts fast. Push the window longer if hunger doesn't hit hard.

Why: Longer fasting deepens fat adaptation and trains mental toughness.

Food:

- ▸ Protein: 200–220g.
- ▸ Carbs: 50–75g. Focus on clean fuel (fruit before training, rice or oats post-training).

Eliminate mindless snacking. Every bite is intentional.

Why: Food is fuel. Nothing more. Nothing less.

Movement: 60–90 minutes daily. Alternate days between cardio focus (5 miles walking/running) and strength focus (bodyweight or weights).

Why: Longer cardio burns more fat. Strength builds your engine. Together, they make you unstoppable.

Tracking: Record your weight and waistline every 3 days.

Why: Proof on paper builds proof in your head. Numbers don't lie.

Mindset Drill: Visualize the man or woman you're building. Write down 3 actions today your old self would've skipped, and celebrate them.

Mantras for Phase 3:

▸ *Proof stacks higher than doubt.*
▸ *Traction > Motivation.*
▸ *As long as it takes. In it to win it.*

By Day 30, the war isn't over, but you'll be unrecognizable compared to the soldier who started. You'll have proof in your body, your mind, and your spirit.

The Rules of Engagement

1. **No cheats.** One soda or one binge can reset momentum.
2. **No negotiations.** Don't argue with yourself. The war plan is law.
3. **No waiting.** There is no "perfect day." There is only today.

Motivation sparks. Discipline sustains. Traction wins.

The War Cry

The next 30 days will not be easy. They're not supposed to be.

But if you execute this war plan without compromise, you'll come out stronger, leaner, sharper, and more dangerous.

Stack your proof. Burn your excuses. The war begins now.

CHAPTER 4

Protein or Nothing

Every diet has its gimmick. Low carb. Low fat. Juice cleanses. Keto. Paleo.

Forget all of it.

If you strip everything else away, the one non-negotiable is protein.

You can eat less and lose weight. Anyone can. But without protein, you'll look like a smaller, weaker version of the same person. You'll burn muscle instead of fat. The number on the scale will drop, but your reflection won't change.

Scale weight doesn't build confidence. Protein does.

Why Protein Wins Every War

Protein isn't just food. It's the raw material for your body's armor. Your muscles. Your hair. Your skin. Your hormones. Your metabolism.

Muscle Preservation: When you cut calories without protein, your body eats its own muscle. That's why crash dieters end up soft, not strong.

Fat Loss: Protein has the highest thermic effect. That means your body burns calories just breaking it down. You're literally torching fat while digesting.

Satiety: Protein kills cravings. A high-protein meal keeps you full hours longer than carbs or fats.

Metabolism: Muscle burns calories even at rest. The more lean tissue you build and protect, the more your body becomes a fat-burning machine.

Protein isn't optional. It's the foundation.

No protein, no progress.

How Much Protein Do You Need?

Forget generic diet charts. Forget "percentages." Here's the battlefield math:

- **Base it on your goal weight, not your current weight.**
- **1–2 grams of protein per pound of goal body weight.**

Example: Goal weight = 180 lbs → 180–200g protein daily.

This isn't complicated. If you want to look strong, lean, and defined, you eat protein like your life depends on it. Because it does.

The Wrong War: Eating Less vs Eating Right

Anyone can eat less and watch the number on the scale drop. But that doesn't mean you win.

Two people can both lose 30 pounds:

- One eats high protein, preserves muscle, and looks leaner, sharper, more powerful.
- The other eats low protein, burns muscle, and ends up smaller but softer, weak, flat, and disappointed when the mirror doesn't match the scale.

The lesson is simple: scale weight means nothing without composition. **It's protein that forms the body you want.**

Weight loss without protein is just self-destruction in disguise.

How to Hit Your Numbers

The excuses end here. It doesn't matter if you're on the road, on a budget, or in the middle of chaos. Hitting your protein is non-negotiable.

Battlefield Foods (No Excuse List):

▶ Chicken breast, lean beef, turkey, fish.

▶ Eggs and egg whites.

▶ Nonfat Greek yogurt, cottage cheese.

▶ Protein powders (whey, casein, plant-based).

▶ Jerky, tuna packets, canned chicken.

Tips to Dominate Protein:

▶ Eat protein at every meal, no exceptions.

▶ Front-load your day: get half your protein in by lunch.

▶ Carry protein with you. Jerky, shakes, bars, always prepared.

▶ Track it. If you don't measure, you won't hit it.

Fail to prepare, prepare to fail.

Protein = Proof

Every pound of fat I lost, every mile I marched, was built on protein. It wasn't carbs. It wasn't hype. It wasn't gimmicks.

It was the discipline to hit my protein numbers every single day, no matter what.

That's why by three months, I didn't just lose weight. I looked like a different man. My body was carving itself into the man I was becoming.

Protein is the proof your body shows the world.

The Test

For the next 30 days:

- ▶ Set your goal weight.
- ▶ Multiply it by 1–2 grams.
- ▶ Hit that number every single day.

No excuses. No exceptions.

Eat your protein, or stay the same.

The War Cry

The scale can lie. Fatigue can lie. Excuses will always lie.

But protein never lies. It builds you from the inside out.

Protein or nothing. That's the only way forward.

CHAPTER 5

Grams Don't Lie

Numbers don't care about your feelings.
The scale doesn't care about your excuses.
And food doesn't care about your intentions.
That's why you measure. Always.
Because grams don't lie.

The Problem With Guessing

Most people think they can eyeball their food. A scoop of rice. A handful of chips. A splash of oil.

Wrong.

- That "serving" of peanut butter you eyeballed? It's probably double.
- Those "21 chips" the bag calls one serving? Grab a handful and you're over by 100 calories without even noticing.
- That restaurant salad they claim is 600 calories? Try 900 or 1000.

When I first bought a digital food scale, I thought I was eating "one scoop" of peanut butter a night. When I measured it, I found out it was almost three. That was over 400 calories I didn't even realize I was adding.

A few bites here, a few sips there, and suddenly your "deficit" is gone. You're not burning fat — you're maintaining or even gaining.

Eye-balling is lying.

Why Grams Win

When you measure in grams, there's no room for error. No "about." No "close enough."

▶ Grams tell the truth about calories. One extra spoon of rice? Measured.

▶ Grams tell the truth about protein. 100g of chicken breast ≈ 31g protein.

▶ Grams keep you honest. No more "that looks like a serving." You know.

Two extra spoonfuls of peanut butter a day = 200 hidden calories. Multiply that by 30 days and you've eaten 6,000 calories you didn't account for. That's nearly two pounds of fat — gained by accident, just from guessing.

Full accountability = full control.

This is why soldiers inventory gear piece by piece. Because when your life depends on it, guessing isn't an option. Your war with food is the same.

The Restaurant Trap

Restaurants aren't built to help you. They're built to keep you coming back.

That "healthy bowl" with "half a cup of rice"? More like a cup and a half.

That "6 oz steak"? It's a mystery how much butter and salt they add each time.

That "light dressing"? It's dumped with a ladle.

You're not eating what you think you're eating. You're eating what they gave you.

That's why the only meals you can trust are the ones you weigh yourself.

Control what you can control. Don't outsource discipline.

Why "Servings" Lie

Food companies print labels to look friendly, not accurate.

▶ "One serving = 21 chips." But no two chips weigh the same.

▶ "One scoop protein powder = 30g." But one scoop packed heavy might be 40g, one loose might be 25g.

▶ "One serving cereal = ¾ cup." What does that even mean? Cups aren't precision. Grams are.

The only number that matters is the one on the scale. Not the back of the box.

Labels round. Grams count.

The Discipline of Weighing

You don't weigh food because you're obsessed. You weigh food because you're in a fight.

A soldier counts bullets before a mission. You count grams before a meal. Both are survival.

And it's simple:

▶ Buy a digital scale.

▶ Weigh everything before you eat it. Meat, rice, oats, peanut butter, even chips.

▶ Log it. Track it. Own it.

At first, it feels slow. But in weeks, it becomes automatic. In months, it becomes freedom.

Because when you weigh your food, you know your numbers. And when you know your numbers, you control your outcome.

Discipline isn't obsession. Discipline is freedom.

No Room for Error

The reason most people fail isn't lack of effort. It's lack of accuracy.

They think they're in a deficit, but they're not.
They think they're eating enough protein, but they're not.
They think "close enough" counts, but it doesn't.

When you weigh your food, you eliminate error. You eliminate lies. You eliminate excuses.

If you're not measuring, you're guessing. And if you're guessing, you're losing.

Your Mission

- ▶ Buy a food scale today.
- ▶ Weigh everything you eat for the next 30 days. No exceptions.
- ▶ Record it. Protein, carbs, fats. Every gram.

You'll be shocked how far off you've been. And once you see the truth, you can never unsee it.

Grams don't lie. People do.

The War Cry

The battlefield doesn't care about your estimates.

The mirror doesn't reward "about right."

And your body doesn't run on intentions.

It runs on grams.

Measure everything. Own everything. Because grams don't lie.

CHAPTER 6

MTKU: Move to Kill the Urge

The battlefield doesn't wait for perfect conditions. Cravings don't care if you're tired, stressed, or already crushed under the weight of life. They ambush you. They whisper lies. "Just one won't hurt. You've earned it. Tomorrow you'll start again."

This is where most people lose.
This is where I refused to die.
I created a rule. A command. A weapon.

MTKU: Move to Kill the Urge.

The Rule of War

Every time a craving hit, I didn't negotiate. I didn't sit there and let the thought marinate.

I moved.

Push-ups.

Sit-ups.

Marching in place.

Jogging to the mailbox and back.

It didn't matter what the movement was. What mattered was that weakness never got the final word.

The second the urge arrived, I killed it with sweat.

Weakness doesn't get a vote.

But it does get a funeral.

Why It Works

Movement floods your body with endorphins. It resets the brain. It takes the urge, the storm of chemicals screaming for sugar, soda, or comfort food, and drowns it under blood flow, oxygen, and adrenaline.

Your brain can't hold two battles at once. When you're gasping for air mid-push-up set, the urge loses its grip.

Science backs it. Psychology confirms it. But more than that, I lived it.

Example: The Candy Bar War

Picture this: you're standing in the gas station staring down a Snickers bar.

250 calories of weakness.

One bad decision that can undo hours of discipline.

Here's the MTKU rule:

Instead of buying it, step outside and march hard for 15 minutes.

Result? You burn roughly the same 250 calories while killing the urge.

The craving dies, the proof stacks, and you walk away stronger than when you walked in.

Weakness starves. Discipline feasts.

Example: Liquid Landmines

Cravings don't just come wrapped in candy bars. Sometimes they show up in a bottle.

A 20-ounce soda? **250 empty calories.**

That fancy coffee drink? **400+ calories of sugar and cream disguised as "energy."**

Even so called "healthy" smoothies can pack over 500 calories of blended sabotage. Shakes can add **1,000-plus calories.**

That's half a day of discipline destroyed in a few gulps.

Here's the MTKU response:

Before you drink weakness, earn strength.
Drop and give yourself 25 push-ups.
Go walk hard for 10 minutes.
Make your body sweat before your mouth decides.

Nine times out of ten, the urge dies before the drink ever hits your lips.

And if you still choose to drink it? At least you've forced yourself to weigh it against the cost.

Every sip has a price. MTKU makes you pay in proof, not excuses.

Making Urges Work for You

Here's the truth: urges never go away. You don't outgrow them.

But with MTKU, you turn every urge into an alarm.

Instead of "I want sugar," it becomes:

"I get to earn another rep."

Instead of "I want comfort," it becomes:

"I get to sharpen my edge."

The enemy thinks it's ambushing you, but every attack just makes you stronger.

Sacred Discipline

When I moved to kill the urge, I wasn't just fighting food cravings.

I was rewiring my identity.

From man of excuses to man of execution.

From "I can't resist" to "I don't negotiate."

From consumer to conqueror.

Every urge became an invitation to stack proof.

Your Orders

From this chapter forward, you don't let urges win.

You don't "resist." You attack.

The rule is simple:

If the urge shows up, you move. Immediately.

It can be ten push-ups.

It can be a walk to the end of the block.

It can be air squats until your legs burn.

Doesn't matter what it is, what matters is that weakness learns one lesson:

You hit back harder.

The Truth

Motivation won't save you here.

Discipline will.

MTKU isn't theory. It's a battlefield tactic. It will work for anyone, anywhere, anytime.

Not because it's fancy, but because it's ruthless.

Step after step. Rep after rep. Craving after craving.

Move to kill the urge. Kill it before it kills your progress.

CHAPTER 7

Steps = Sanity

Discipline doesn't always come with fireworks. Sometimes it comes one foot in front of the other.

When I was losing weight, I discovered something that changed everything: **steps kept me sane.**

Calories burned, cravings crushed, stress reduced, all of it came back to movement.

The more I walked, the more my mind cleared. The more I tracked my steps, the more control I felt over the chaos.

Steps weren't about being fancy. They were about being consistent.

Why Steps Matter

Everywhere you go, your body keeps score. You're either stacking proof with movement or stacking excuses with inactivity.

Think about this:

- **10,000 steps** is about five miles.
- At an average pace, that's **400–500 calories burned.**
- Do that daily and you're burning an extra **3,000+ calories a week.** That's almost a pound of fat without changing anything else.

But it's more than math. Steps are medicine. They reduce stress hormones. They regulate blood sugar. They keep your joints alive. And they give you proof every single day that you showed up.

When life feels overwhelming, steps simplify everything.

They whisper: "Just keep moving."

From Chaos to Control

I used to drown in noise, cravings, stress, doubt. The weight of life pressed down on me.

But when I stepped outside and started walking, something shifted. My head cleared. The fog lifted. Every step was like clearing debris off the battlefield.

You don't need a gym. You don't need a coach. You don't even need perfect weather. You just need your legs and the will to move them.

That's why I call steps "sanity." They're the reset button you can hit anytime, anywhere.

The Non-Negotiable Baseline

I created a rule: **10,000 steps every day. No excuses.**

Didn't matter if it was raining. Didn't matter if I was tired. Didn't matter if I'd already worked out.

The steps got done. Period.
Why? Because I knew this:

Food can lie. Scales can lie. Steps don't lie.

If I hit my step count, I could trust my discipline was intact.

Some days I pushed harder and hit 20,000. Other days I had to grind late at night in the dark to get my last 2,000. But I never let the counter rest below 10,000.

That baseline kept me sharp. It gave me a number I couldn't negotiate with.

How to Hit Your Sanity Steps

Here's the battlefield playbook:

▶ **Start Early.** Knock out 2,000–3,000 steps before noon. It builds momentum and keeps you from scrambling at night.

▶ **Stack Movement.** Walk while you're on calls. Park farther away. Take stairs instead of elevators. Steps hide everywhere.

▶ **Break It Down.** Don't think 10,000. Think 1,000 at a time. Mailbox to mailbox. Block to block. Lap to lap.

▶ **Track Ruthlessly.** Use a phone, watch, or pedometer. Don't guess. Guessing is lying. Numbers are proof.

▶ **Use Steps as Urge-Killers.** (MTKU in motion). When cravings hit, walk until they die.

The Mind Game

Steps aren't just physical. They're psychological.

The act of walking forward tells your brain you're moving toward something better. It's symbolic. It's momentum in its rawest form.

When you're stressed, angry, or tempted —> walk.

When you're doubting yourself —> walk.

When you're ready to quit —> walk.

I walked through blizzards in Chicago. I walked laps around my driveway in Florida humidity. I walked at midnight under streetlights when everyone else was sleeping.

Each time I finished, I felt peace. The chaos didn't own me anymore.

Steps equal sanity.

Example: Stress vs. Steps

One night I came home from a brutal day. Stress was screaming at me to binge. The fridge was calling my name.

Instead of cracking open the food, I laced up my shoes and started walking. One lap. Then another. Then another.

By the time I hit 3,000 steps, the urge was gone. My stress was sweating out of me instead of eating into me.

If I had given in, I'd be stacking regret.

Instead, I stacked proof.

Sacred Simplicity

We all want complex programs. Secret hacks. Fancy formulas.

But here's the truth: **sometimes sanity is as simple as steps.**

Every step is proof. Every step is momentum. Every step is discipline in motion.

You don't need to run a marathon. You don't need to be perfect. You just need to keep moving.

Brick by brick. Step by step. Proof by proof.

Marching Orders

From this chapter forward, steps are no longer optional.

They're the baseline. The sanity line.

- **10,000 a day minimum.**
- Track it.
- Hit it no matter what.

When the chaos comes, when the cravings hit, when the doubts scream, move your feet.

Because if you can walk, you can win.

Bottom Line

Motivation won't get your steps in.

Discipline will.

And once you learn to walk through the chaos, you'll never lose your sanity again.

Steps = Sanity.

CHAPTER 8

Sleep Debt = Snack Debt

You can run on fumes for a while. You can grind through exhaustion and push your body past its limits. But eventually, if you don't pay your sleep debt, your body will charge you interest — and that interest is hunger.

I learned the hard way: every time I cut sleep, I craved trash. Chips. Candy. Fast food. Soda. The weaker my sleep, the stronger the cravings.

That's why I call it sleep debt = snack debt.

If you owe your body hours of sleep, you'll pay it back with calories you never needed.

The Battlefield of Hormones

This isn't just willpower. It's chemistry.

- **Sleep deprivation spikes ghrelin** — the hunger hormone. That means every food commercial, every smell from a drive-thru, every thought of sugar feels 10x stronger.
- **Sleep deprivation drops leptin** — the hormone that tells you you're full. That means even after eating, you don't feel satisfied.
- **Lack of sleep also raises cortisol** — your stress hormone. And cortisol screams for comfort food.

Studies show that just one bad night of sleep can lead to **eating 300–400 extra calories the next day.** Multiply that by a week of poor sleep, and you've overeaten the equivalent of an extra **1–2 pounds of fat.**

You're not weak when this happens. You're human. Your biology is stacking the deck against you.

That's why discipline isn't just about food and steps. It's about sleep.

The Domino Effect

One bad night of sleep doesn't just make you tired. It wrecks your whole day.

- You skip your morning workout because you're exhausted.
- You drink three cups of coffee, each loaded with sugar or cream.
- You snack mid-morning because you're dragging.
- You overeat lunch because your hunger signals are broken.
- You hit the afternoon crash and raid the pantry.
- By night, you're so depleted you either binge or say, *"I'll start over tomorrow."*

All from one missing block of sleep. That's the domino effect of sleep debt.

My Rule: CPAP + Curfew

I used to stay up late scrolling my phone, eating snacks in front of the TV, telling myself "just one more hour." But those hours cost me weeks of progress.

So I built non-negotiables:

- **Bed by 9 p.m.**
- **CPAP strapped on.**
- **Kitchen closed by 7 p.m. sharp.**

That routine saved my life. It cut my cravings in half. It gave me back energy for my workouts. And it stacked proof while everyone else was still bargaining with themselves in the fridge at midnight.

Example: The Midnight Raid

Before I locked in, I'd fall into what I called the midnight raid. I'd be dead tired, lying in bed, and suddenly my brain would whisper: "Go grab something from the kitchen. Just a little snack."

That "snack" turned into 500–1,000 calories in the dark. Chips, ice cream, soda. Empty proof that erased the work I'd done earlier.

Now? The kitchen is a battlefield with a locked gate. When 7 p.m. hits, the war is over. No late-night raids. The line is drawn.

Sleep as a Weapon

Most people treat sleep as a luxury. Something extra. Something you'll catch up on later.

But if you want to win the war against weakness, you need to treat sleep as a weapon.

- Sleep sharpens discipline.
- Sleep repairs muscles.
- Sleep balances hormones.
- Sleep makes cravings weaker.

Sleep is strategy. Lack of sleep is sabotage.

Hack: Power Naps

Sometimes life won't let you get 7–8 hours at night. Work, kids, stress — it happens.

That's where power naps come in. **15–20 minutes max.** Enough to recharge your brain without leaving you groggy.

It's not a replacement for deep sleep, but it's a battlefield tactic when you're under fire.

Steps + Sleep = Sanity Multiplied

Remember Chapter 7? **Steps = sanity.**

Well, here's the multiplier: when you combine steps with quality sleep, your discipline becomes unstoppable. Your cravings drop. Your stress lowers. Your metabolism runs hot.

That's why I tell people:

▶ Steps during the day protect your sanity.
▶ Sleep at night protects your discipline.

Together, they're armor you can't afford to take off.

Your Move

From this chapter forward, you fight sleep debt like you fight sugar. Because every hour you lose is another urge waiting to ambush you.

▶ **Set a curfew.** Don't negotiate.
▶ **Strap in.** If you need CPAP, use it every night. No excuses.
▶ **Lock the kitchen.** No food past your cut-off.
▶ **Prioritize 7–8 hours.** Guard it like your life depends on it — because it does.

The Last Mile

Sleep debt equals snack debt.

You either pay with hours in the bed or with pounds on your body.

Discipline doesn't just live in the gym or at the dinner table. It lives in the dark, when nobody's watching, when your only job is to rest.

Protect your sleep. Protect your progress. Protect your proof.

CHAPTER 9

Starve The Traps

Weakness doesn't just live inside you, it lives around you.

In your pantry. In your fridge. In the break room. On billboards. In drive-thrus waiting to ambush you.

Everywhere you go, traps are set.

Sugar. Salt. Fat. Quick comfort. Easy dopamine.

But here's the rule of war: **you can't negotiate with traps. You have to starve them.**

The Trap Game

The food industry is a battlefield designed against you.

- ▶ The bright packaging.
- ▶ The buy-one-get-one deals.
- ▶ The "family size" bag that's secretly meant for one sitting.
- ▶ The "healthy" label slapped on sugar bombs.

These aren't mistakes. They're weapons.

Their goal is to keep you hooked, eating more, and coming back for another round.

And if you keep weakness within reach, eventually weakness will win.

That's why my rule became simple:

If it's a trap, it doesn't live in my house. Period.

My Early War with Traps

At my heaviest, I used to keep Oreos, chips, soda, and frozen pizza in the kitchen. I told myself, *"I'll just have one. I'll control it this time."*

That "one" turned into a binge every time.
The problem wasn't willpower. The problem was proximity.

In fact, studies show that when food is within arm's reach, people eat up to **70% more** than when it's stored just a few steps away. Environment matters more than intention.

So I stripped the battlefield.

- No soda in the fridge.
- No chips in the pantry.
- No ice cream in the freezer.

If I wanted to binge, I'd have to drive to the store. That extra barrier killed the urge 90% of the time. By starving the trap, I starved my weakness.

Build the War Zone

You can't just avoid traps, you need to **fortify your territory.**

Here's the playbook:

- **Pantry audit:** Throw out every trigger food today. Not tomorrow. Today.
- **Fridge reset:** Fill it with lean proteins, vegetables, fruit, and water. If it doesn't build discipline, it doesn't belong.
- **Car sweep:** Fast food wrappers, energy drinks, candy — clear it out. Your car is either a weapon or a weakness.
- **Work zone control:** Keep healthy snacks or protein shakes at the office. Don't rely on the vending machine to fuel your proof.

Every environment you control either stacks discipline or stacks temptation. Make your environment your ally, not your enemy.

Example: The Gas Station Trap

You stop for gas. You walk inside. The smell of pizza. The glow of candy bars. The coolers packed with soda.

That's a trap.

Here's the tactic: don't go in. Pay at the pump. Reframe the battlefield. You're there for fuel, for your car, not your body.

If you must go in, go in with a shield: buy water. Walk out. Nothing else. No negotiation.

Every avoided trap is proof stacked. Every surrender to a trap is proof burned.

Food Isn't Love

One of the deadliest traps is emotional eating. Celebrations, comfort, boredom. We tie food to every emotion.

But food isn't love.

Food isn't comfort.
Food isn't stress relief.
Food is fuel. Nothing more. Nothing less.

Once you sever that lie, you take power back. Weakness loses its weapon.

The Illusion of Moderation

Most people will tell you, "Everything in moderation."
That's another trap.

Moderation sounds wise. It sounds balanced. But here's the truth: if moderation worked for you, you wouldn't be at war with your body.

Moderation is weakness with better branding.

Discipline means knowing which traps you can never negotiate with.

For me? Soda, fast food, desserts. I cut them out cold turkey. I didn't manage them. I buried them.

You don't moderate poison. You eliminate it.

Starve the Traps, Feed the Proof

Every trap you remove is one less ambush.
Every weakness you starve is one more brick of proof stacked.

At first, it feels harsh. Like you're cutting out all the fun. But what's fun about being weak? What's fun about hating the mirror? What's fun about living trapped by cravings?

Starve the trap, and you starve the old version of you.
That's the war you're fighting.

The Code

From this chapter forward, you live by this code:

- ▶ If it's a trap, it doesn't enter your home.
- ▶ If it's a trigger, you cut it off completely.
- ▶ If it weakens you, you don't negotiate — you starve it.

Build a war zone that stacks discipline. Create an environment where proof wins and weakness dies.

Because traps only have power when they're fed.

Final Word

Motivation won't save you when there's ice cream in the freezer.

Discipline will.

Starve the traps, feed the proof.

And watch the old you die of starvation.

CHAPTER 10

Travel, Parties, Pressure: Still in Control

Travel, holidays, business dinners, weddings, these are the battlefields where habits die.

Lights, drinks, social pressure, unfamiliar food, disrupted sleep: it's the perfect ambush. Most people surrender. They tell themselves, "I'll start again when I'm back." Then they come home with proof burned and regret stored.

Not you. Not anymore.
You don't avoid the world. You bring the war with you.
You win the mission wherever you land.
Still in control. Always in control.

The Mindset Before You Leave

Every successful operation starts with a plan. Travel and parties are no different.

Before you step out the door, declare your non-negotiables. Not fuzzy goals. Not "I'll try." Real rules:

- **Protein first.** (I carry protein in the plane, in the car, in my bag.)
- **Fasting window locked.** (Use flight or event time to cover your fast.)
- **Step baseline.** (I hit X steps every day even on vacation.)
- **No traps allowed.** (Soda, fast food, dessert? Not in my immediate supply chain.)

Write this down. Put it on your phone as an alarm. Make it your war brief. When pressure shows up, you fight for the rules you set before you left.

If it's not in the mission brief, it doesn't happen.

Travel Tactics (Planes, Trains, Cars)

Travel is chaos. Use the chaos to your advantage.

1) Pack a Travel Arsenal

Bring the tools that make discipline non-negotiable:

▶ A travel protein kit (3–4 single-serve protein powders or high-protein bars, jerky packets, tuna packs).

▶ A small canister of instant oats and a scoop (if you need solid morning fuel).

▶ A collapsible water bottle.

▶ A resistance band and a compact towel.

▶ A sleep mask + earplugs and your CPAP if you use one.

▶ Phone charger, schedule screenshots, and your "mission card" with a 1-sentence reminder of why you're doing this.

Pro tip: airline delays are predictable, so is hunger. Your kit makes you unpredictable to cravings.

2) Use Travel Time as Fasting Time

Flights, layovers, and long drives are perfect fasting windows. Eat before you go (protein heavy). Lock 14–16 hours. By the time you land, you'll be eating on your schedule, not the airport's.

3) Eat Before You Board, Not Onboard

Airport food is a trap. If you must eat in the terminal, stick to grilled chicken salad (dressing on the side), a hard boiled egg pack, or that protein kit. Avoid snack bars and high sugar bakery items.

4) Hotel Room Warfare

You don't need a gym. You need a plan:

- **Bodyweight circuit:** 5 rounds: 20 body squats, 10 push-ups, 15 glute bridges, 30-second plank. 20 minutes and you've killed an urge and stacked proof.
- **Morning walk:** 30–60 minutes outside before the day starts. It resets circadian rhythm, reduces jet lag, protects sleep.
- **Request a mini fridge:** stash protein items and water. Hotel coffee is filler and expensive, plan your real fuel. *(Don't rely on someone else for your health)*

5) Jet Lag = Tactical Opportunity

Use light exposure, steps, and a fast to reset. Arrive in daylight, walk 10-12k steps, and force yourself into the local schedule. Don't nap more than 20 minutes unless it's a survival move. Sleep when the battle demands it, but win the day.

Win the Room Without Losing the War at Parties & Social Events

Parties are engineered to make you snack, drink, and forget your plan. Don't let them.

1) The Arrival Strategy

- Eat a protein-rich snack before you go. You won't be clinging to bread while you mingle.
- If it's an event with a buffet, stand opposite the spread, position matters. The further you are from the food, the less likely you'll pile a plate in one motion.
- Hold a drink that isn't calorie-packed (sparkling water with lime). People think you're drinking; you aren't sabotaging your war.

2) The Social Script (Say it Like a Soldier)

You'll get pressure. Have short, polite, non-negotiable scripts:

- ▸ "I'm on a challenge; I'll pass tonight."
- ▸ "I'm driving tomorrow, so just water for me."
- ▸ "I ate already; I'm just here for the company."
- ▸ "I'm good, appreciate it though" (sometimes the simplest responses are best, you owe nobody a explanation)

People accept short, confident answers. No excuses. No justifications. Don't debate. Command.

3) The Plate Strategy

If you're handed a plate:

- ▸ Fill half with protein (meat, fish, eggs).
- ▸ Fill one-quarter with vegetables.
- ▸ Fill one-quarter with carbs if performance demands it.
- ▸ Skip the breadbasket. Skip the seconds. One round only.

4) The Drink Strategy

Alcohol is the easiest sabotage. Use strategies:

- ▸ Alternate every alcoholic drink with a water.
- ▸ Choose lower-calorie options: spirits with soda water, wine (dry), light beer.
- ▸ Pre-commit: "Two drinks only," and switch to water.
- ▸ Or: skip alcohol altogether and own the night. You'll remember the fight, and results in the morning.

5) Bring Your Own Backup

If appropriate, bring a healthy dish. It's a stealth move. Everyone eats your food, and you control one corner of the battlefield. For work events, this is often acceptable; for private parties, it's a power move.

Business Dinners & Pressure: Still in Command

Business meals are high stakes, they mix relationship pressure and rules. But influence doesn't require surrender.

1) The Pre-Game Brief

▶ Eat protein before the meeting. If you arrive full of protein, you won't be tempted by breadbaskets.

▶ Scope the menu online. Pick your options in advance to avoid impulse decisions under pressure.

2) Order Like a General

▶ Appetizer: protein (oysters, shrimp cocktail, chicken skewers).

▶ Entrée: grilled meat, fish, or a steak. Ask for sauces on the side.

▶ Sides: vegetables, baked potato (if needed). Skip fries.

▶ Dessert: decline politely. "I'm sweet enough; thank you." If they insist: the table shares, remember it's not rude to put your health first."

3) The Negotiation Script

If coworkers insist on a second bottle or dessert: use short commands:

▶ "I'm sticking to my plan tonight."

▶ "I appreciate it, but I'm not drinking tonight."

▶ "I've got an early flight, I'll pass."

Assertive, not apologetic. Respect earns respect.

Genius Tactics You Won't Hear at a Seminar

You asked for tactics that aren't common, here are the ones that actually flip the field.

1) The "Mission Card" Carry Your Why

Write a 1 sentence mission on an index card: "14-16 hour fast, 200g protein, 10k steps." Put it in your wallet. Pull it out when pressure comes. It proves you planned. It's harder to sabotage yourself when your why is literal paper in your hand.

2) The "Kitchen Lock" Hotel Edition

For longer trips, buy a small, travel combination lock and secure a suitcase of non-perishables in the closet of your room. It sounds dramatic and it is, but your discipline will thank you when temptation is out of arm's reach.

3) The "Pocket Scale" Trick

Bring a small digital scale. Weighing restaurant portions is a power move. Yes, people will think you're odd. So what? You're not here for applause, you're here to win.

You're not trying to be like everyone else, stop trying to fit in.

4) The "Pre-Order + Confirm" Move

For business lunches, pre-order your meal online for pick up and ask the restaurant to hold sauces. You show up with your plate pre selected and no awkward decision making under pressure.

Tip: You can get food with oils, salt, butter. All restaurants will do this!

5) The "Report Back" Accountability Text

Before an event, text your red wire (wife, friend, coach): "On mission. I'll report back at 10 p.m." Send a photo of your plate or your step count. Public accountability spikes compliance.

6) The "Time Shift Trick"

If an event is late-night and you know it breaks your fast, shift your eating window earlier that day. Cover the event's time with a longer fast before. You win the timing, you don't let the party set your clock.

Sleep, Steps, MTKU Bring Your Weapons Everywhere

Don't drop the fundamentals because you're traveling. The war plan travels with you.

- ▶ Sleep: maintain curfew where possible. Use masks and earplugs. If you lose a night, power nap.
- ▶ Steps: schedule morning walks; make sightseeing your cardio.
- ▶ MTKU: urges will appear amplified on trips; respond with movement immediately. Use hotel stairs, parking lot laps, and resistance bands.

When you maintain the basics, everything else becomes easier.

Contingency Plans (Because Life Breaks Plans)

No plan survives contact without a backup. Here are contingency plays:

- ▶ **If you miss your fasting window:** accept it, lock the next window, and double down on protein. No guilt. No reset culture. Proof stacks forward, not backward.
- ▶ **If you overindulge:** don't binge on guilt. Do MTKU immediately. Walk, move, and return to plan at the next meal. One mistake isn't surrender, it's intelligence if you correct fast.
- ▶ **If social pressure is relentless:** leave early. Your mission matters more than one night of social approval. Leave with dignity and proof.
- ▶ **If your luggage is lost:** use local grocery stores. Tuna packets and rotisserie chicken exist everywhere. Be resourceful.

Closing: Command the Room, Don't Be Commanded By It

Travel and parties aren't interruptions to growth; they're tests of it. Most people let the world run them. You don't. You plan, you pack, you pre-commit, and you execute. You bring your weapons: protein, steps, sleep, MTKU, and the mission card.

If you follow this chapter, you'll return from every trip intact, maybe even better. Proof stacks while others burn it.

You go where life takes you, but you bring the war with you. Still in control. Always in control.

CHAPTER 11

Proof Over Plateaus

Every soldier in this war will hit a wall.

The dreaded plateau.

The scale freezes. The mirror doesn't move. The progress feels stuck. And your brain whispers: "Why bother? It's not working anymore."

That's the ambush. That's the illusion.

And here's the truth: **if you're doing everything right, there is no plateau.**

The Lie of the Scale

The scale doesn't measure discipline.

The scale doesn't measure proof.

The scale doesn't know about your sleep, your steps, your protein, your fasts, your resistance against cravings.

It only measures gravity. And gravity can lie.

Your body isn't a math problem on a bathroom floor. It's a battlefield of hormones, muscle, water, glycogen, and proof. The number may hold steady, but proof never does. Proof stacks daily.

That's why you never let the scale define your mission.

Proof Over Plateaus

When the number stalls, here's your checklist of proof:

- ▸ **Steps:** Are you hitting your baseline every day? (10k+ minimum.)
- ▸ **Protein:** Are you locking 1–2 grams per pound of goal weight? No excuses.
- ▸ **Fasting window:** Is your daily fast intact? No snacks sneaking past the lines?
- ▸ **Food measured:** Are your grams logged with precision? (No eyeballing, no "close enough.")
- ▸ **Sleep:** Are you banking 7–8 hours with curfew and CPAP?
- ▸ **MTKU:** Are you killing urges with movement instead of feeding them?
- ▸ **Environment:** Have you starved the traps? No poison in the pantry?
- ▸ If these are stacked, if every one of these proofs is intact, then the plateau doesn't exist. You are winning, period. The mirror will catch up. The scale will break eventually.

The War Against Illusions

Your body plays tricks on you. Water retention. Hormonal shifts. Muscle gain while fat loss continues. Stress levels. Sodium spikes.

In fact, studies show most people can retain 2–5 pounds of water weight in a single day from stress, high sodium meals, or hormonal shifts. That has nothing to do with fat gain, it's just your body holding water like a sponge.

That's why plateaus aren't real, they're illusions created by short term noise.

When I was down 100 pounds, the scale stalled for nearly two weeks. I was ready to rage. But when I reviewed my proof. Every fast locked, every mile run, every gram measured. I realized the mission was intact. The illusion broke. Within another week, the scale dropped 7 pounds overnight.

That wasn't magic. That was proof over plateaus.

This Is the A-Z Route

You don't take detours in this war. There are no pit stops at "maybe." No resting at "good enough."

This is the **A-Z route.**
You start at A. You finish at Z.
No stopping at B. No bailing at C. No sightseeing at M.

Proof is the straight line through the alphabet. Plateaus are the letters trying to distract you. Ignore them. Keep marching.

Example: The Soldier's Ruck

Think of a soldier on a ruck march. Pack on his back. Miles ahead.

He doesn't stop because the terrain looks the same for an hour. He doesn't quit because the GPS doesn't show progress every step. He keeps walking. Step after step. Proof after proof. Until the destination appears.

Plateaus are like flat terrain. They feel endless. But *if you're stacking proof, you're still moving forward. The destination is guaranteed.*

No Room for BS

This chapter cuts all excuses.

- ▶ If you're eyeballing food, that's not proof.
- ▶ If you're skipping steps, that's not proof.
- ▶ If you're half fasting, that's not proof.
- ▶ If you're sleeping 5 hours and calling it discipline, that's not proof.

Plateaus are only real if you're lying to yourself. If you're following the mission with zero cracks, then the plateau is nothing but noise.

No BS. No excuses. Only proof.

The Proof Test

Here's how you kill the doubt:

At the end of each day, run the Proof Test. Ask yourself:

- ▶ Did I hit my steps?
- ▶ Did I crush my protein?
- ▶ Did I respect my fast?
- ▶ Did I measure every gram?
- ▶ Did I protect my sleep?
- ▶ Did I move to kill urges?
- ▶ Did I starve the traps?

If the answer is YES across the board, then you are winning. No matter what the scale shows.

Doors are shut.

From this chapter forward, plateaus don't exist in your vocabulary. The scale is background noise. Proof is the only scoreboard.

Stack the proof. Review the proof. Trust the proof.

Because when the war is fought with discipline, the body has no choice but to surrender.

Lock it in

Plateaus are illusions. Proof is real.

If you're doing everything right: every step, every gram, every hour of sleep, every urge killed, every trap starved, then you are winning. Period.

This is the A-Z route. No stops at B or C.

You march until you finish.

Proof over plateaus. Always.

CHAPTER 12

Lose Loose Skin

Everyone fears it.
Loose skin.

It's the ghost hanging over every weight loss journey. People whisper about it in forums, DM about it in secret. They'll take any excuse not to start because, deep down, they're not just afraid of failing. They're afraid of succeeding and looking in the mirror at a body they don't recognize.

But here's the truth:

Loose skin is not a reason to quit.
Loose skin is not punishment.
Loose skin is proof.

The Test

I want you to stop reading for a second and take this test. When I say:

"Loose skin is 50% genetics."

What's your first thought?

"I knew it. I have bad genetics. Why even try? I don't want to lose weight and end up with loose skin."

Or

"Okay, 50% genetics. That means 50% lifestyle and habits. That's my lane. That's my battlefield. That's where I win."

Right there is the real battle.

The difference between excuse and execution.

Life gives you a million reasons why not. You only need one reason why to.

The Science Experts Don't Talk About

Even most "experts" don't fully understand loose skin. They talk about it like it's a punishment for losing weight. But here's what they miss:

Collagen production declines with age, stress, and poor nutrition. Muscle loss under the skin accelerates sagging.

Hydration, protein, and micronutrients fuel the skin's repair process as much as your muscles.

Inflammation and hormones determine how elastic your skin stays during weight loss.

You can't change your genetics. But you can absolutely control the environment your skin is healing in.

High protein = building blocks for collagen.
Resistance training = keeps lean mass under the skin.
Hydration and micronutrients = skin elasticity.
Avoiding ultra-processed food = lower inflammation.

Most people don't even know these levers exist. They just give up before they start. But not you. You're reading this. That already puts you ahead.

Mindset > Excuses

Here's the truth: your body isn't punishing you. It's adapting. Loose skin isn't a flaw. It's evidence you've escaped a trap that almost killed you.

You can see it as a badge of shame or a badge of honor. That's your choice.

When people DM me, "Cristian, what about loose skin?!" I ask them one question:

"Would you rather live another decade at 300+ pounds, or wear a little proof of your victory?"

That question changes everything.

The Curveball Story

Things won't just come easy. Life will always throw curveballs. They come fast, they come hard, and they almost always arrive when you least expect them. The curveball doesn't ask if you're ready. It doesn't care if you're standing tall or already stumbling. It just comes.

The only thing that matters is how you react, how you adjust, and whether you're willing to step back into the batter's box after you've already been knocked down.

I learned that the hard way on the night I lost everything.

I came home to find a pink slip waiting for me. Fired. Just like that, the last bit of stability I had left evaporated. No savings. No backup plan. That job was my rope, and it had snapped.

I drove to Walmart to buy a cheap pillow, because I already knew where I'd be sleeping. My car was about to become my bed, my closet, my kitchen, and my home. I told myself it was temporary. But when I walked out into that dimly lit parking lot, pillow under my arm, my car wasn't there. Gone. Repossessed.

I stood there stunned, staring at an empty parking space like it might magically fill itself again. In a single day, I'd lost my job and my car. I had no money, no home, no backup plan, no options. Just a pillow I didn't even need anymore.

I walked. Not because I had anywhere to go, but because walking was the only thing that still moved when my life didn't. My feet carried me to the one place that felt familiar: my old high school bleachers. I climbed the cold metal, stretched out, and stared up at the stars. I had never felt smaller, more disposable, more irrelevant.

In my pocket was a sheet of LSD. A literal exit. I thought, Why not just take it all? Nobody would care.

My phone buzzed. It was my mom. She didn't argue. She just stayed on the line a little too long, her silence heavier than words. And that silence cracked something open in me.

I hung up, stared across the empty field. And that's when I saw it. The school's digital billboard lit up across the parking lot:

"Looking for a better path? United States Navy."

I don't believe in coincidences. I believe in crossroads. Acid in one pocket. A billboard in my line of sight. Death on one side. Life on the other.

I pocketed the acid. I picked up my phone. I made a choice. That same night, I reached out to a Navy recruiter and started my journey back.

That night didn't fix everything. But it did one crucial thing: it snapped me awake. It reminded me that I had a choice, even when it didn't feel like I did.

And years later, when I was 370 pounds staring at the scale, I remembered that choice. Because my addiction to food, to comfort, to escape, it was the same acid in my pocket. Another slow exit. And I decided, Not today. Not anymore.

How This Applies to Loose Skin

Loose skin is your acid test.

It's the moment you decide whether you'll let fear stop you or proof drive you.

You can't control your genetics. But you can:

Lose weight at a steady pace (no crash dieting).
Train your muscles under the skin (resistance training).
Stay hydrated and nourish your body (collagen, micronutrients, healthy fats).

Use natural methods to help lymphatic drainage and skin tightening. (I practice what I teach, my own methods helped me minimize loose skin dramatically.)

Do all this, and your loose skin may be dramatically less than you expect. Even if it's not perfect, it will be a thousand times better than living sick, heavy, and trapped.

A Mindset Flip That Changes Everything

Loose skin isn't a reason not to lose weight. It's a reason to do it right. It's a reason to fight harder. It's proof of your freedom. And freedom looks better with a little battle damage than chains ever will.

Life will hand you curveballs. Genetics will hand you curveballs. The question isn't whether the pitch is fair. It's whether you swing anyway.

Because one day, you'll look in the mirror at skin that's not perfect but a life that's yours. You'll realize you're not just lighter. You're alive.

Your Turn

Stop using loose skin as an excuse.
Start using it as fuel.
Control what you can: protein, hydration, training, micronutrients, sleep.

Accept what you can't: genetics, age, scars.
You're not chasing perfection. You're chasing freedom.

And freedom always beats fear.

Lock It In

The scoreboard won't care how smooth your skin looks. It will care that you showed up, swung anyway, and built a life worth living.

Loose skin isn't the enemy. Excuses are.

And when you finally strip the weight, the old habits, the old story, you'll realize something: you were never fighting loose skin. You were fighting yourself. And you won.

Loose Skin, Quick Fixes, and the Hard Truth

Most people want to believe the lie: there's an easy way out.

I believed it too. I spent years searching for shortcuts, gadgets, and miracle fixes. And every time, the truth hit me harder:

There are no quick fixes. Not for fat loss. Not for loose skin. Not for life.

Yes, you have to work hard to lose the weight. But here's the kicker: it's even harder to lose weight and not have loose skin. That's the next level of discipline. And that's why so many people quit before they ever start, they already believe the lie that they're doomed no matter what.

The secret isn't finding a magic solution. The secret is accepting the hard road and walking it anyway.

Why Hard Is the Point

If there was a pill that burned fat, tightened skin, and sculpted abs overnight, would you even be proud of it? No. Because the value is in the fight.

That's the paradox: the struggle is the gift. Loose skin is the reminder. The hunger pangs, the sore muscles, the setbacks, they're not obstacles. They're the training ground.

Life doesn't reward easy. Easy gives you diabetes, regret, and broken promises. Hard gives you freedom.

Quick Fix Culture: The Modern Trap

Look around today. Semaglutide. Ozempic. Wegovy. Weight loss "miracle shots."

They're marketed like salvation. But what nobody tells you is this:

the shot can shrink your appetite, but it can't fix your habits.

It can't teach you how to choose protein over pizza.

It can't teach you to walk mailbox-to-mailbox until you can run five miles.

It can't teach you to stack proof when motivation dies.

And here's the brutal truth: people taking these quick fixes often end up with the worst loose skin. Because they dropped weight without building lean muscle, without feeding their skin, without creating habits that keep them whole.

The shot ends. The habits never formed. The weight comes back. And the shame deepens.

My Desperation for a Shortcut

I get it. I've been there.

At one of my lowest points, I started chasing treatments. I researched liposuction, CoolSculpting, body contouring, anything that might give me the look I wanted without the grind.

That's when I found Laser Fat Loss. Non-invasive. "Safe." Promising to melt the fat away.

I drove to a facility in Poway, California. The building looked like a spa, fountains outside, crisp clean smell inside. The woman behind the desk smiled, pinched my love handles, and said words that hooked straight into my insecurity:

"We can fix that."

She wrote up a $1,400 package. I hesitated. She pressed harder. Logic slipped. I called Kenzie. She wanted me to feel better in my own skin, so she said yes.

I left with "hope." I left with ten sessions.

For ten weeks, I followed their program: water intake, steps, clean food. I did it all. At the end?

I had gained 10 pounds. Added 7 inches.

My stomach dropped. Fourteen hundred dollars. Ten weeks of effort. And the result was worse than when I started.

When I confronted her, she smiled and said, "You just need more packages."

It was like being sold poison after you'd already been poisoned. I walked out defeated, depressed, and broke.

That moment broke me harder than the scale ever did.

The Uniform Story: When Shame Shows Up Everywhere

Back in the Navy, weight wasn't just my private battle, it was public humiliation.

Uniform inspections every morning. Regulations so strict you couldn't hide a wrinkle, let alone a belly. As I ballooned in weight, I had to custom-order uniforms because stores didn't even stock my size. Belts didn't exist for me. I taped mine together with double-sided tape, just to fake the look of compliance.

I had one uniform left that fit. I never washed it because it was the only one. It stank. The armpit stains never came out. The blouse buttons strained so hard I had to leave two undone just to breathe.

That was my reality. Living proof that chasing quick fixes instead of facing the truth doesn't just cost you money. It costs you dignity.

The Truth About Loose Skin and Fixes

Here's what I learned the hard way:

Loose skin is 50% genetics. You don't control that.

The other 50% is lifestyle. Protein. Hydration. Resistance training. Micronutrients. Sleep. Skin elasticity is not random. You can influence it.

But no laser. No shot. No wrap. No gimmick will ever replace the daily habits that train your body to heal while it transforms.

Loose skin is the receipt of your victory. But how that receipt looks depends on whether you paired fat loss with habits that nourish your skin as much as your muscles.

Accepting the Hard Way = Accepting Freedom

I want you to pause here. Because this is the fork in the road.

You can chase the illusion of easy. You can spend money on injections, treatments, surgeries, and still end up broken, scarred, and disappointed.

Or you can accept the hard way. You can embrace the reality that there are no shortcuts worth taking. And in that acceptance, you will find freedom.

Because the real "fix" is not in skipping the pain. It's in surviving it.

The Power of Process

When I finally stopped chasing treatments and accepted the grind, everything changed. I leaned into the long days, the endless measuring, the moments I hated the mirror.

And somewhere along the way, I learned the secret:

The process is the point.

The suffering is what strips you down. The discipline is what builds you up. The proof stacks, mile after mile, meal after meal.

That's why my skin didn't collapse the way I feared. Because while I was losing fat, I was feeding skin, feeding muscle, feeding my body the tools to heal.

And even if genetics had given me the worst-case scenario, I would have worn my scars like a badge of honor. Because scars mean you lived. Scars mean you fought. Scars mean you won.

Where Quick Fixes Really Lead

Think about it:

A shot won't raise your daughter.
A laser won't stop your cravings.
A surgery won't teach you how to stack proof.

Those things can change a body. But they can't change a life.

And if you don't change your life, the body always bounces back to where it was.

That's why you can't chase fixes. You have to chase freedom.

Because no quick fix will leave a permanent change.

Who's Next

If you're afraid of loose skin, let me leave you with this:

Loose skin means you lived. Loose skin means you didn't quit. Loose skin means you swung the bat when the curveball came.

But loose skin isn't the end of the story. With the right habits, you can minimize it, tighten it, and adapt your body to a new life.

And more importantly, you'll realize the battle was never about skin. It was about excuses. And you've already proven you can kill those.

So choose the hard way. The lasting way. The real way.

Because freedom doesn't come from shortcuts. It comes from scars.

CHAPTER 13

Protein vs. "Protein"

Everyone says they eat protein.
But not all protein is created equal.

There's a massive difference between real, whole protein and the processed protein impersonators that flood shelves today.

You can't shortcut this war. Your results depend not just on eating protein, but on the source.

Why Protein Matters

Protein isn't just "muscle food." It's survival food.

▶ Repairs tissue.
▶ Builds lean mass.
▶ Fuels recovery.
▶ Produces neurotransmitters that affect mood, sleep, and focus.

When I dropped 200 pounds in a year, protein was my anchor.

It wasn't carbs. It wasn't fat. It was protein.

Without it, the weight would've melted the wrong way: weak, sagging, burned out. Instead, I stayed lean, strong, and disciplined.

Whole Protein vs. Processed Protein

Here's the truth most people don't want to hear:

Protein shakes, bars, and powders are last-resort survival rations.

Whole proteins: chicken, beef, fish, eggs, Greek yogurt. These are your real ammunition.

Yes, Quest bars and powders carry protein grams on the label. But they also carry fillers, gums, and sweeteners that confuse your body. That's why so many people who live off them feel bloated, sluggish, and still hungry.

I know because I abused them. I leaned on bars and shakes as "anchors" instead of last resorts. I thought I was dieting at 300 pounds while chugging Atkins shakes, pounding Quest cookies, and drinking my calories down. But instead of losing weight, I gained more. I didn't understand that "protein" wasn't the problem, fake protein was.

When I finally went to war with myself, I cut all that noise. My foundation became whole protein, specifically chicken tenderloins and everything changed.

Now? I only touch powders or bars when I'm traveling, fasting 24+ hours, and I'm literally choosing between that or fast food. That's the only time. Never as a foundation.

The Chicken Truth

From nearly 400 pounds down to 170, chicken was my mainstay. Plain, repeatable, disciplined.

Why chicken?

Lean: High protein, low fat.

Healing: Packed with amino acids that repair tissue, support skin, joints, and recovery.

Mood: Contains tryptophan, a precursor for serotonin — your "feel better" chemical. Protein stabilized my brain as much as my body.

Proof: I ate chicken every day and stayed lean while losing 110 lbs in 90 days, 150 lbs in 5 months, and 200 lbs in a year.

People ask if I got bored. The truth? Boredom is what made me obese.

I chased pleasure with food.

Discipline made me free.

Superfoods in the Mix

I'll be real: I hate avocado. The texture, the taste. Just not my thing.

But I still ate it. Why? Because it's a superfood.

Avocado is loaded with:
Healthy fats for hormone balance.
Potassium for recovery.
Fiber for digestion.

And here's the key: you don't need buckets. A little every day stacks up more than a mountain once in a while.

Note: Superfoods aren't about what you like. They're about what works.

Processed vs. Ultra-Processed vs. Whole

To make this crystal clear, here's the battlefield breakdown:

Whole Protein:

Chicken, beef, fish, eggs, plain Greek yogurt.
Minimal ingredients. Maximum benefits.

Processed Protein:

Greek yogurt with flavoring, rotisserie chicken with seasoning, jerky with additives.
Still useful, but less clean.

Ultra-Processed Protein:

Protein bars, powders, Quest, shakes with fillers, gums, preservatives. Emergency rations only. Never your foundation.

The Math of Protein vs. Junk

Back when I was obese, I'd down pasta, soda, and breadsticks in one sitting 4,000–6,000 calories easy. But I wasn't nourished. I wasn't full.

On my war plan, I ate more food than ever: chicken, rice, spinach, avocado. Huge plates. Loaded bowls. Clean, measured, whole. I was eating more volume than ever but fewer calories.

Tip: A serving of chicken tenderloins (4 oz) = 24g protein, 110 calories. That means 1 lb of chicken = 440 calories, 96g protein. That's one of the most powerful macro weapons on earth.

Protein fills. Heals. Rebuilds. Junk just weighs you down.

Why Grams Matter Here Too

Eyeballing is lying. Labels can mislead. Grams don't lie.

- A "scoop" of powder? Depends on humidity, settling, scoop size. Not accurate.
- A "bar" with "20 grams protein"? That's on the label, not in your absorption. Whole food wins.
- A "chicken breast weighed raw at 200g"? That's truth. That's proof.

Grams don't lie. Labels do.

Non-Negotiable: Protein From the Right Source

This is why my war worked. My proof wasn't just about calories, it was about quality. Every gram counted. Every bite was stacked for victory.

Your body becomes what you feed it:

▶ Junk in = broken body.
▶ Proof in = proof out.

Whole protein is proof.
Processed protein is survival rations.
Ultra-processed protein is enemy propaganda.

Your Move

Here's the creed:

▶ Build your diet on whole protein.
▶ Use processed sparingly.
▶ Reserve ultra-processed for emergencies only.
▶ Add superfoods daily, even in small doses.
▶ Remember: it's not about less food. It's about better food.

If you want your war to end in victory, your body must be rebuilt brick by brick.

And the bricks are protein.

Lock It In

Protein isn't negotiable. The type of protein isn't negotiable.

I didn't lose 200 pounds by chasing shortcuts. I lost it by locking in whole protein, every day, without fail.

Powders and bars may trick the masses. But not you. Not now. Not ever.

Protein is proof. The new you demands it.

CHAPTER 14
Hungers Psychology

Hunger Is Not the Enemy

Most people think the enemy is hunger.
Every ad you've seen says it: "Suppress your appetite." "Crush your cravings." "Never feel hungry again."

Pills. Shakes. Shots. Gimmicks. They all paint hunger as the villain.
But let me break the truth to you: hunger is not the enemy. Hunger is the test.

Hunger is a signal, nothing more. It tells you something is happening inside your body. Sometimes it's real. Sometimes it's fake. Most people can't tell the difference.

When I was nearly 400 pounds, I swore I was hungry all the time. Morning, night, in between meals. I thought it was endless. But looking back? Most of it wasn't hunger at all. It was boredom. Stress. Addiction. Habit.

The problem isn't hunger. The problem is how you've been trained to answer it.

The Two Hungers

Here's the truth: there are only two types of hunger.

1. Physical Hunger (Body Hunger)

This is real. It builds slowly. You feel it in the stomach, emptiness, rumbling, maybe some fatigue. It's solved with fuel: protein, hydration, nutrients.

2. Psychological Hunger (Mind Hunger)

This is fake. It hits suddenly, like a sucker punch. Triggered by emotions, commercials, the smell of popcorn at the movies, or scrolling Instagram food reels. It's solved not by food, but by awareness and discipline.

Here's the part that hurts: 90% of the hunger people feel isn't real.

Most of what you call hunger is just your brain looking for dopamine.

And if you don't know the difference, you'll feed both, and stay stuck.

The Hunger Test

I'll give you a weapon right now.
When hunger strikes, do this:

- ▶ Drink 16 oz of water.
- ▶ Wait 15 minutes.

If it's still there, it's body hunger. If it fades, it was fake.

That simple.

I call it the Hunger Test. Do it every time, and you'll start realizing how many lies you've been swallowing.

Hunger as Addiction

Hunger feels urgent because it's tied to survival. Your brain is wired to respond to it like an emergency. The same dopamine circuits that fire for drugs and gambling fire for food.

That's why chips don't just taste good, they light your brain up like a slot machine. That's why soda doesn't just quench thirst, it delivers a dopamine hit that leaves you chasing the next sip.

Your hunger isn't broken. It's hacked.

And just like any addiction, you don't fix it with shortcuts. You fix it by rewiring the system.

Hunger Comes in Waves

Here's what I learned from fasting: hunger is not a straight line. It doesn't just keep building until you collapse. It comes in waves.

And like waves, they crash and pass.

The first time I realized this, it changed everything. I thought if I didn't eat, the hunger would just keep climbing until I broke. But then... it faded.

That's when I understood: hunger is not a command. It's a suggestion.

The weak follow it. The disciplined ride the wave until it breaks.

Hunger Isn't a Signal to Eat. It's a Signal to Lead.

Every time my stomach growled, I reframed it. Instead of hearing, "Eat," I heard, "Train."

Growl? That's another pushup.
Craving? That's another sprint.
Mind says quit? That's another mile.

Discipline is built in the moments nobody sees. Hunger gave me those moments every day.

When I stopped seeing hunger as punishment and started seeing it as proof, I became unstoppable.

The Science of Hunger

Let's get tactical.

Hunger is not random. It's hormones. And if you don't understand the chemistry, you'll keep thinking your willpower is the problem.

Ghrelin: The hunger hormone. Spikes before meals. Drops after. If you train your body to expect food every 2–3 hours, it will spike constantly. If you eat on a set schedule, you train ghrelin to behave.

Leptin: The satiety hormone. It tells your brain when you're full. Obesity wrecks leptin. Your body stops hearing the signal. The only fix? Lose fat slowly and restore sensitivity.

Insulin: Manages blood sugar. Every soda, breadstick, or candy bar spikes insulin, leading to crashes that mimic hunger. That's why you feel "hungry" an hour after fast food.

Most people don't have a hunger problem. They have a hormone problem.

And hormones reset with consistency, not diets, not shots, not pills.

Hunger and Volume

I eat more food now than I did at 370 pounds. The difference? The volume is clean.

Then:

Pasta, soda, breadsticks. 4,000–6,000 calories in one sitting.

Now:

2–3 pounds of chicken, lean beef, rice, spinach, avocado. Massive bowls, huge plates, half the calories, ten times the fuel.

That's the cheat code: eat more, eat smarter.

Lean protein first. Grams don't lie. Hunger gets crushed, discipline gets built.

Quick Fixes Are Poison

I've seen the hype around weight-loss shots, fat-freezing, body sculpting. Everyone wants the shortcut.

But here's the truth: shortcuts don't teach discipline.
Weight-loss shots? Kill your appetite short-term, but destroy muscle and leave you with loose skin.

Fat-freezing? Attacks the surface but does nothing for hormones, habits, or discipline.

Powders and pills? Just ways to avoid facing the truth: you eat too much and move too little.

Quick fixes numb hunger. They don't master it. And when the fix runs out, the hunger comes back stronger.

The secret isn't avoiding hunger. It's conquering it.

Hunger in the Field

There were nights I thought my hunger would break me. Days when I'd worked out for hours, fasted 16–18 hours, and my body screamed.

But here's the phrase that saved me: hunger is temporary, regret is permanent.

If I gave in, I'd feel good for five minutes and hate myself for five days. If I pushed through, I'd feel proof for a lifetime.
That's the exchange: five minutes of pleasure or a lifetime of pride.

Hunger and Identity

The most powerful shift you'll ever make is identity.

Most people lose to hunger because they see themselves as people who "eat when hungry."

The new you says: "I'm not the kind of person who folds at the first pang."

That identity shift makes hunger powerless. You stop fighting cravings as battles and start living as someone who doesn't negotiate with weakness.

Weapons Against Hunger

Here are the exact weapons I use:

16 oz Water Rule – Hunger gets water first. Fake hunger dies fast.

Protein First Rule – Protein kills fake hunger and keeps you full longer than carbs or fat.

Move Rule (MTKU) – Craving? Drop for pushups, walk, do burpees. Hunger dies when you move.

Routine Rule – Eat at the same times. Train ghrelin to obey you.

Sleep Rule – 7–9 hours. Sleep debt makes hunger hormones go wild.

Delay Rule – Push every craving 10 minutes. Most vanish before time is up.

These aren't tips. These are orders. You follow them or you fail.

Hunger Is Proof

Here's the secret nobody tells you: if you never feel hungry, you're not losing fat.

Hunger is proof you're in the fight. Hunger is proof you're breaking old patterns. Hunger is proof your body is adapting.

Every stomach growl is a receipt of progress. Every craving denied is another brick stacked.

Hunger means you're winning.

The Psychology of Hunger: Beyond Food

Hunger doesn't just hit your stomach. It hits your mind.

It says: "You can't do this. You'll always be fat. You'll always cave."

But here's the twist: hunger is the perfect metaphor for life.

In business, hunger is that urge to quit when sales dry up.
In relationships, hunger is the craving for comfort instead of growth.
In life, hunger is the voice telling you to settle instead of fight.

If you master hunger here, you master it everywhere.

A Story of Hunger Training

At 370 pounds, I couldn't walk a block without gasping. My stomach growled constantly. I thought it was proof I was broken.

So I tested it. I went for 24 hours without food. Just water, black coffee, and sheer will.

The hunger came in waves. Morning was brutal. Afternoon worse. Evening nearly broke me.

But then, midnight came. The hunger faded. I wasn't dead. I wasn't even weak. I was alive, and stronger than I'd ever felt.

That was the night I learned hunger is a liar. It tells you you'll die if you don't feed it. But if you stand tall, it bows down.

Hunger and Loose Skin

Here's where it ties back: hunger isn't just about weight. It's about the skin you wear after.

Crash diets, quick fixes, and fast drops? They shred muscle and collagen, leaving you with loose skin.

Disciplined hunger management, protein, resistance training, hydration, micronutrients build lean tissue under the skin, supports elasticity, and gives your body a fighting chance to tighten.

Master hunger, and you master not just fat loss, but skin survival.

Hunger and Freedom

At my heaviest, I was chained by hunger. Every craving, every pang, every urge dictated my life.

Now? I'm free. Not because hunger disappeared, but because it lost its power.

I still feel it. I still get cravings. But I don't answer them with excuses anymore.

That's the freedom you're chasing: not smaller pants. Not a lower scale number. Control.

Your Mission

Stop fearing hunger.
Use it as training.
Rewire your hormones with discipline.
Build meals on lean protein and whole food.
Sleep, hydrate, move, measure.
Stack proof every time you deny a craving.

Final Word

Hunger is not punishment. Hunger is proof. Hunger is the forge where the old you burns away and the new you is built.

You don't need to numb it. You don't need to fear it. You need to master it. Because the warrior who can stare hunger in the face and keep marching is the warrior who wins.

Hunger is your battlefield. Master it, and you master yourself.

CHAPTER 15

Chakra Energy

Most people have heard the word "chakra" tossed around in yoga classes, self-help books, or even wellness conversations. To someone new, it might sound mysterious, mystical, or even unbelievable. I get it, I used to feel the same way.

But here's the truth: when you strip away the surface layer of spiritual vocabulary and look at the concept through history, psychology, and biology, chakras can be understood in a way that makes practical sense even if you don't believe in "energy healing."

This chapter is not about convincing you to adopt a belief system. It's about giving you a framework that connects body, mind, and perception. Whether you see chakras as energy centers or simply as a map for self-awareness, they can give you clarity on how to live a stronger, more aligned life.

What Are Chakras?

The word chakra comes from Sanskrit, an ancient Indian language, and literally means "wheel" or "disk." In spiritual traditions like yoga, tantra, and Ayurveda, chakras are described as spinning centers of energy that run along the spine and influence physical, emotional, and mental well-being.

The traditional framework identifies seven main chakras:

1. Root (Muladhara) – survival, safety, stability.
2. Sacral (Svadhisthana) – sexuality, creativity, pleasure.
3. Solar Plexus (Manipura) – willpower, confidence, digestion.

4. Heart (Anahata) – love, compassion, balance.
5. Throat (Vishuddha) – communication, self-expression.
6. Third Eye (Ajna) – intuition, focus, insight.
7. Crown (Sahasrara) – consciousness, meaning, spirituality.

From a spiritual perspective, when these centers are open and balanced, life force (prana) flows freely. When blocked, it creates imbalance.

Now, that's the traditional story. But what if I told you there's also a scientific bridge here, one that makes chakras relevant even to the most skeptical reader?

The Nervous System and Chakras

One way to translate chakras into science is through the nervous system, particularly the autonomic nervous system, which regulates unconscious processes like breathing, heartbeat, digestion, and stress responses.

The root chakra, at the base of the spine, sits where the spinal cord connects to the pelvic nerves, which handle survival instincts like fight-or-flight.

The sacral chakra is near the reproductive organs and sacral plexus nerves that influence sexuality and bladder function.

The solar plexus chakra overlaps with the celiac plexus, nicknamed the "abdominal brain," a hub of nerves that controls digestion and stress.

The heart chakra aligns with the cardiac plexus, a nerve cluster around the heart that regulates heart rate and emotional states.

The throat chakra connects to the cervical ganglia and thyroid gland, which regulate metabolism and voice.

The third eye chakra links to the pineal gland and hypothalamus, brain centers tied to hormones, circadian rhythms, and intuition.

The crown chakra has no direct organ but is associated with the cerebral cortex, the seat of higher thought and awareness.

So while chakras are not literal glowing wheels, they map surprisingly well to real biological hubs where nerves, hormones, and emotions intersect.

The Psychological Lens

Here's another way to look at it. Chakras can also serve as a psychological model of human development and motivation.

The root chakra resembles Maslow's "physiological and safety needs."

The sacral chakra relates to relationships, intimacy, and creativity.

The solar plexus chakra matches self-esteem and personal power.

The heart chakra ties to belonging and love.

The throat chakra reflects communication and authenticity.

The third eye chakra mirrors insight and foresight.

The crown chakra resonates with self-actualization and meaning.

Even without any spiritual belief, chakras give us a map of human needs and growth. Coaches, therapists, and leaders often use this language because it resonates with people. For example, someone with trouble speaking up may be told their "throat chakra" is blocked. Whether you take that literally or not, it's pointing to a real pattern: difficulty with expression.

The Endocrine Connection

Science also gives us a biological link: the endocrine system, which controls hormones. Each chakra corresponds to a gland:

▸ Root – adrenal glands (stress response).
▸ Sacral – reproductive glands (sexual hormones).

- Solar plexus – pancreas (digestion, insulin).
- Heart – thymus (immune system).
- Throat – thyroid (metabolism).
- Third eye – pineal gland (sleep/wake cycles).
- Crown – pituitary gland (master regulator of hormones).

Ancient yogis didn't know anatomy in modern terms, but through meditation and self-observation, they mapped patterns that align closely with what science has confirmed.

Why Chakra Practices Work

Whether you believe in energy flow or not, the practices associated with chakras: meditation, yoga, breathing, chanting, are proven to change your body and mind.

- Meditation calms the nervous system and lowers cortisol.
- Breathwork activates the parasympathetic system, reducing stress.
- Yoga postures open physical areas tied to each chakra.
- Chanting stimulates the vagus nerve, improving relaxation.
- Visualization activates imagination centers in the brain, influencing mood and motivation.

So, even if you ignore the word "chakra" entirely, these practices still produce measurable results.

Caution and Criticism

Now, let's be clear: chakras are not physical organs. You can't dissect a human body and find them. They are metaphors and experiential maps.

Some scientists dismiss them as pseudoscience. Others see value in them as tools for self-reflection and mental regulation. The placebo effect itself proves that belief shapes physiology.

The danger is in going too far, thinking chakra balancing alone can cure cancer or replace medical treatment. That's not reality. But as a complement to science-based health, chakras offer a powerful perspective.

Why They Still Matter

Here's why chakras remain relevant today:

1. They unify body and mind instead of splitting them into separate boxes.
2. They give us a language of self-awareness that's simple and relatable.
3. They connect to validated practices like meditation and breathwork.
4. They mirror the journey of human growth, from survival to purpose.

My Take – A Root Chakra Lesson

For me, the study of chakras is amazing because it reveals something deeper: what we look for is what we find.

I've lived this lesson through the root chakra, the one tied to survival, safety, and stability.

There was a time when I was under crushing stress, financially strapped, bills stacked high, my mind racing with the thought that my wife might leave me. I felt like the floor could drop out from under me at any second. That's what a blocked root chakra feels like: fear, insecurity, instability.

But then something shifted. I took a step back and asked myself: Has she left yet? Have I lost the roof over my head yet? The truth was, no. None of those fears had become reality. And I realized I had been lower before, and survived. That thought hit me like a lightning bolt: if I had been lower, then the only direction left to go was up.

That's the power of perception. Nothing outside of me changed in that moment, my bank account didn't magically refill, my circumstances didn't immediately improve, but my focus did. Instead of obsessing over what could go wrong, I saw what was still right. Instead of sinking into fear, I found strength in perspective.

That's what chakras, whether you view them as energy centers or metaphors, remind me of: your brain is your perception. Every thought, every focus, every story you tell yourself shapes the reality you experience.

The real challenge isn't memorizing the seven chakras or trying to keep them perfectly balanced. The challenge is learning to control and own your perception. Balance isn't about invisible energy alignment, it's about choosing how you interpret your world. It's about refusing to let fear and old patterns dominate you.

When you take responsibility for your perception, you stop reacting to life and start creating it. And that is what true balance looks like.

Challenge Time

So here's the question I'll leave you with:

Are you willing to take ownership of your perception, your focus, and your energy, and use it to build the life you know you're capable of?

Because science shows the body and brain are deeply connected. Chakras give us a language for that connection. And your mindset, the way you choose to perceive reality is the lever that determines whether you stay stuck or step into possibility.

What once felt mysterious and mystical is now practical. It's not about glowing wheels of energy. It's about perception, focus, and growth. It's a roadmap you can choose to walk every single day.

Energy Walks In First

The first thing that walks into a room isn't your words.

It's your energy.

I learned that lesson in the Navy. The kind of place where weakness doesn't hide, it's exposed under fluorescent lights and echoing metal walls. One morning, I walked into the training room with my nerves on fire. My heart was racing, chest tight, every breath shallow. My jaw locked so hard it ached. I didn't have to say a word; everyone felt it.

The instructor didn't even look at me before barking, "Lopez, get your head right."

He didn't need to see my report, he could feel my chaos.

That's when it hit me: people don't just hear you, they read you.

They feel your state before you ever speak. The nervous twitch in your leg, the breath stuck in your throat, the stiffness in your shoulders, it all speaks louder than your voice ever could.

Energy isn't mysticism. It's biology.

Stress leaks through your breath, posture, and tone. It's chemistry screaming through body language.

And for most of my life, that energy was running me.

When Stress Ran My Life

Years later, I was no longer in uniform, but my body was still in battle.

I was 370 pounds. Overworked, under-slept, juggling family, bills, and the kind of silent panic that follows you into bed at night.

Every morning, I'd wake up with my heart pounding like I was late for a fight.

But there was no fight, just a flood of cortisol and adrenaline.

My breath never made it past my chest.

I confused anxiety for hunger. I fed panic instead of peace.

I didn't realize it then, but I was carrying loud stress energy everywhere I went.

People could sense it, the tension, the rushed words, the weight behind my smile.

When your nervous system is at war, everyone around you feels the blast radius.

It wasn't until I started studying the connection between breath, biology, and presence that I saw the truth:

Your body doesn't lie. And if you don't control your energy, it will control you.

The Science Behind Energy

Let's strip the fluff. Energy isn't "vibes." It's biochemistry.

When you're stressed, your brain floods your system with cortisol and adrenaline. Your breath shortens. Your heart rate spikes. Blood leaves your organs and rushes to your limbs for survival. You stop thinking long term and start reacting.

That's not spiritual, it's survival programming.

Now, ancient cultures described this same biological system through chakras, energy centers in the body.

Modern science calls them nerve plexuses and endocrine hubs.

Different language, same truth.

▸ Root Chakra – Safety. Biology: adrenals, cortisol.
▸ Solar Plexus – Willpower. Biology: blood sugar, insulin.
▸ Heart Chakra – Connection. Biology: heart rate, oxytocin.
▸ Throat Chakra – Expression. Biology: breath, vagus nerve.

The deeper you breathe, the more you regulate every one of them. The shallower you breathe, the more chaos you create.

Quick test:

Right now, place a hand on your chest and one on your stomach. Which moves when you inhale?

If it's your chest, you're breathing stress. If it's your belly, you're breathing power.

Stories of Breath That Saved Me

The Navy Drill

Under pressure, I discovered something called box breathing-inhale four, hold four, exhale four, hold four. At the time, I thought it was just a focus trick. Turns out, it was chakra alignment in disguise. It grounded my root, stabilized my heart, and pulled me out of panic.

The Weight Loss War

When I started losing weight, I realized half my "hunger" was anxiety. I'd take a deep breath instead of reaching for food, and suddenly, the craving vanished. Hunger was just stress wearing a mask.

The Stage Moment

Years later, standing before an audience, I felt my throat tighten, the old nerves. I slowed my breath, grounded my feet, inhaled deep into my stomach. The crowd didn't change, but my energy did. Suddenly, they leaned in. Presence replaces panic every time.

Chakras Demystified

Forget crystals and incense. Chakras are your body's energy checkpoints, where emotion meets biology.

- Root (Safety): I remember waking up in my car once, broke, exhausted, and humiliated. No safety, no stability. My root collapsed. That's when I learned: safety isn't money. It's self-trust.
- Sacral (Emotion): I used to numb feelings with food and noise. When I stopped suppressing emotion, energy started to flow again.
- Solar Plexus (Willpower): Every skipped workout, every broken promise to myself weakened this center. Consistency rebuilt it.
- Heart (Love): I shut people out when I felt shame. Love can't breathe through armor.
- Throat (Expression): The first time I spoke about my struggles publicly, I felt my throat unlock. Truth heals faster than silence.

Reset tools:

- Breathe into discomfort.
- Journal what you won't say out loud, or write in phone notes.
- Move your body daily.
- Ground yourself barefoot on earth.

You can't meditate your way out of misalignment, you must move energy through the body that created it.

The Cortisol Cycle You Must Break

Here's the loop that destroys millions of lives:

Stress $\rightarrow$ Shallow breath $\rightarrow$ Cortisol spike $\rightarrow$ Fat storage $\rightarrow$ Cravings $\rightarrow$ Guilt $\rightarrow$ More stress.

You snack after bad news. You yell at your kids for nothing. You scroll instead of sleeping. That's not lack of willpower-it's a hijacked nervous system.

Your body stores fat when it doesn't feel safe.

And safety starts with breath.

Every exhale tells your brain, I'm okay.

Every shallow inhale tells it, I'm under attack.

The moment you break this cycle, your biology realigns with your purpose.

The Breathing Routines That Rebuilt Me

Box Breathing (Navy Roots): Inhale 4, hold 4, exhale 4, hold 4. Builds calm in chaos.

4-7-8 Breathing (Night Anxiety): Inhale 4, hold 7, exhale 8. Knocks out adrenaline before bed.

Power Breaths (Before Battle): Quick, deep diaphragmatic breaths to flood the body with oxygen before workouts or speeches.

Each breath is a reset button for your nervous system, and an alignment tool for your chakras.

Energy in Environments

Energy multiplies or mirrors.

I've walked into rooms carrying heaviness so thick you could feel it in the air. Conversations felt forced. People avoided eye contact.

Later, I learned that when I walked in calm, grounded, and focused, everything shifted. People spoke slower. My kids relaxed. Even the dog settled.

You don't just change rooms by what you say.

You change them by how you breathe.

Routine Is Energy Medicine

Chaos fuels cortisol. Structure stabilizes it.

My old life was unpredictable, random meals, no sleep, zero rhythm. My body never felt safe. Today, everything I do stacks calm instead of chaos:

- ▶ Morning breath-work before phone.
- ▶ Consistent meal timing.
- ▶ Evening wind-down without screens.

Routine is rhythm, and rhythm regulates energy.

You don't need a guru. You need structure.

Because when your days have order, your energy has direction.

Your energy walks in first.

Everywhere you go, your biology speaks before your words do.

So breathe deep. Stand tall. Align before you act.

When your energy leads with calm power, the world listens because you're not just in the room anymore.

You own it.

Create a 7-day Energy Reset:

- ▶ Day 1: Midnight breath audit.
- ▶ Day 2: Root grounding (walk barefoot or lift heavy).
- ▶ Day 3: Solar plexus wins (track & conquer one meal).
- ▶ Day 4: Heart connection (gratitude call).
- ▶ Day 5: Throat expression (say one truth).
- ▶ Day 6: Third eye clarity (10 minutes meditation).
- ▶ Day 7: Crown alignment (revisit your why).

Commanding the Room

I remember the first stage I ever stepped onto.

The weight was gone, but the energy of the man who carried it still lingered.

My body had changed, but my nervous system hadn't caught up yet. The memory of being 370 pounds, ashamed, anxious, and invisible, still lived somewhere in my chest.

When I stood backstage, I could feel him. The old me. The one who used to hide behind food and noise. The one who would've rather disappeared than been seen.

Now hundreds of eyes were waiting for me. Lights blinding, air thick, the low hum of anticipation vibrating through the room.

My heart started to race. That familiar tightness crawled back into my throat. For a second, it felt like I was back in that Navy training room stressed, jittering, chest locked.

But this time, I didn't let it own me.

This time, I moved.

I dropped down for a quick round of jumping jacks right there backstage.

I spoke out loud to myself, direct, commanding, no excuses:

"This is my energy. This is my body. No environment, no person, no situation has the right to own me. I control me."

The crowd's energy was trying to pull me in, but I reversed it.

I took the nerves, the jitters, and turned them into power.

My pulse steadied. My breath deepened.

In that instant, I wasn't a victim of energy anymore, I was its architect.

When they called my name, I walked out slow, deliberate, each step a declaration of ownership.

Every breath grounded.

Every thought clear.

I didn't need to hype myself up or "fake" confidence. I was confidence.

When I reached center stage, I paused, three seconds of stillness that felt like eternity. The entire room leaned in.

Then I spoke. Slowly. Intentionally.

My tone steady, my words precise.

And the moment the sound left my mouth, I felt the energy flip.

The crowd didn't change me.

I changed the crowd.

Every inhale fed my presence.

Every exhale anchored my message.

And standing there, I understood something no book or course could teach:

The strongest man in the room isn't the one flexing force.

It's the one whose energy is mastered.

Presence isn't about dominance, it's about self-command.

It's the quiet signal that says, "I'm here. I'm certain. You're safe to follow."

When I finished, the applause didn't feel like noise, it felt like alignment.

I didn't walk off that stage like a performer who nailed his speech.

I walked off like a man who had finally met himself.

Because for the first time...

I wasn't chasing energy.

I was energy.

Energy walks in first.

And when yours is calm, grounded, and aligned

the world can't help but follow your lead.

Brand this into your brain

- Stress isn't just in your head. It's in your breath.
- Cortisol is the enemy of fat loss, focus, and peace.
- Chakras aren't mysticism; they're body-energy systems tied to biology.
- Breath + routine = your new medicine.
- "Energy doesn't just change you, it changes the world around you."

The Bigger Picture

Life doesn't stop. It doesn't pause when you're tired. It doesn't soften because you've been through enough. It just keeps coming. Problems keep showing up, pressure keeps building, and every day you wake up in a world that demands more from you than you think you can give.

Here's the truth most people never learn: the problems aren't the problem. The problem is focus.

You get what you focus on. You find what you're looking for. And what you say to yourself becomes your truth.

If you keep telling yourself, "I'm stuck. I'm too fat. I'm too broke. I can't win," then congratulations, you just wrote the script for your life. You just programmed your brain to find proof of failure in everything you see.

But shift your focus, even slightly, and the whole picture changes.

Seeing What's Right

It doesn't have to be dramatic. It can be as simple as this: "I can stand on my feet today."

Sounds cliché? Maybe. But think about it. There are people who would give anything just to stand again. To breathe without tubes. To sleep without pain. To walk into their kitchen and pour a glass of water without help.

Gratitude isn't soft. Gratitude is clarity.

Every human rich, poor, successful, broke, lean, obese has problems. But every human also has something good. The difference between those who live and those who just exist is where they put their focus.

If you stare only at what's wrong, you'll find an endless list. But if you shift and start asking, "What's right? What do I still have? What proof do I still control?" then life looks different.

That shift doesn't make problems disappear. But it gives you the strength to face them.

The Silver Lining Rule

I call it the Silver Lining Rule: no matter how bad things get, there's always one thing to hold onto.

You could be broke. You could be homeless. You could be stranded on the side of the road with nothing but this book in your hands. But guess what? That's your silver lining. You've got proof. You're not out of the fight.

Because the fact you're reading these words right now means you're still alive, still breathing, and still capable of gaining traction.

That's the point: any hand can be turned into a winning one. Doesn't matter if it's aces or twos. What matters is how you play it.

Life will always hand you both, reasons to quit and reasons to keep going. Which one you focus on decides who you become.

Why Stress Doesn't Solve Anything

I used to think stress was power. I thought if I worried enough, panicked enough, carried the weight of the world on my shoulders, I'd finally be forced into action.

Wrong.

Stress didn't save me. Stress didn't pay my bills. Stress didn't heal my marriage. Stress didn't burn fat off my body.

All stress did was make me weaker. It ate at me like acid, stripped me of sleep, jacked up my cortisol, kept me bloated, and made me spiral deeper into bad choices.

See, stress isn't a solution. Stress is a magnifying glass. It makes problems look bigger and you look smaller. And when you're trapped under it, you lose sight of what actually matters.

What I needed wasn't more stress. I needed clarity.

Two Questions That Changed Everything

When my world was falling apart, I boiled it all down to two questions. These became my compass:

1. Would my God be proud of me right now?
2. Does this honor my body and the legacy I want to leave?

Those two questions cut through everything.

Now listen maybe your compass isn't God. Maybe it's your family, your kids, your future self. The point is the same: you need a standard outside your excuses to measure against. Something bigger than cravings, bigger than stress, bigger than comfort.

When I asked myself the first question, it pulled me out of selfishness. It reminded me that my choices weren't just mine, they echoed into the people I loved, into the purpose I claimed to live for.

The second question grounded me in reality. Did my choice build me or break me? Did it honor my body or abuse it? Did it move me closer to the man I said I wanted to be, or prove I was still lying to myself?

Once I had that filter, decisions became clear.

Stress was still there. Pressure was still there. But I could finally move forward.

Regret Is the Real Enemy

I can't live with regrets. I can't stomach "what ifs." I can't leave rocks unflipped, doors unopened, chances wasted.

I don't fear failure. I fear reaching the end of my life knowing I never even found out who I could've been.

That's why I push. That's why I show up when it's uncomfortable. That's why I demand the same from you. Because the only way to lose is to quit before you discover your full potential.

No regrets. No what-ifs. That's the mission.

The Bigger Picture in Action

When my marriage was hanging by a thread, when my wife was nine months pregnant and I was overseas, when bills were stacked, when doctors told me I wouldn't make it to 23, the bigger picture was the only thing that saved me.

If I zoomed in on my problems, I was finished. But when I zoomed out, I saw something different: I still had a chance. I still had control over my next choice. I could still fight for my legacy.

That's what I want you to see right now. Your bigger picture.

Maybe you're not at rock bottom. Maybe you're just tired, stressed, stuck in cycles that don't serve you. Doesn't matter. The rule doesn't change:

What you focus on grows. What you say becomes truth.

Start saying something new.

Your Mission

Here's your mission: practice the Bigger Picture Shift every day for the next week.

1. **Morning Focus:** When you wake up, list three things that are right. Doesn't matter how small. Feet on the ground. Breath in your lungs. Kids asleep safe in their beds. Write them down. Speak them out loud.
2. **Midday Reset:** When stress spikes, ask the two questions:
   - Would my God/family/future self be proud of me right now?
   - Does this honor my body and legacy?

If the answer's no, shift immediately.

3. **Night Audit:** Before bed, write one decision from your day that honored your body, and one that didn't. That's your scoreboard. Track it.

Lock It In

The bigger picture isn't about ignoring problems. It's about refusing to let problems own you. It's about seeing what's still good, what's still possible, and what's still within your control.

Stress won't save you. Regret will bury you. Focus will free you.

At the end of it all, you don't want to look back at a life of excuses. You want to look back at proof. Proof that you pushed, proof that you honored your body, proof that you became the person you were meant to be.

So zoom out. See the bigger picture. And then fight like hell to make it real.

Because the truth is simple: every hand can be a winning hand. But only if you play it.

CHAPTER 16

The Days We Don't Want to Show Up

Life Doesn't Stop. Neither Can You.

Here's the first truth: no matter who you are, no matter how disciplined, no matter how motivated, you will face days when you don't want to show up.

And here's the second truth: life doesn't care.

Life doesn't hit pause because you're tired. It doesn't stop because you're hurting. It doesn't slow down because you're behind. Life doesn't ask permission.

Bills keep coming. Pain keeps coming. Hunger keeps coming. Setbacks keep coming.

If life doesn't stop, then neither can you.

The Day the Doctor Said I Wouldn't See 23

At 21, I had the body of a man twice my age, already breaking down.

- Severe sleep apnea.
- Pre-diabetes.
- High blood pressure.
- Nearly 400 pounds of dead weight dragging me toward an early grave.

The doctor didn't sugarcoat it. He said the words flat: "Cristian, we don't see you making it past your 23rd birthday."

Do you think I went home and turned into Rocky that day? Started running stairs and drinking raw eggs?

No. I did what most people do when life punches them in the mouth.

I didn't show up. I drove straight to the nearest fast food place and bought a milkshake.

Because hiding feels good, for five minutes. But hiding doesn't erase the truth.

Not showing up didn't take away the diagnoses. Not showing up didn't stop the scale from climbing. Not showing up didn't protect my future.

It only buried me deeper.

And that's the hard truth most people never admit: not showing up never saves you. It only delays the pain.

The Silent Battles

Everyone loves a transformation picture. The smiling "after" shot. The jeans held out six sizes too big.

But nobody sees the silent battles.

Sitting in the car outside the gym, debating if you'll walk in or just drive home.

Staring at the fridge at 11 p.m., bargaining with yourself about one more snack.

Lying in bed, exhausted, and telling yourself, Tomorrow. I'll start tomorrow.

Those are the battles that matter most. And they don't happen once. They happen every single day.

Transformation isn't built in the big wins. It's built in the moments nobody sees.

Why Showing Up Defines You

It's not about perfection. It's about presence.

The workout doesn't have to be perfect. You just have to show up.

The meal doesn't have to be Instagram-worthy. You just have to stay disciplined.

The day doesn't have to go your way. You just have to face it anyway.

The days you don't want to show up? Those are the days that decide your entire future.

Anybody can show up when it's easy. Winners show up when it's hard.

The Psychology of Quitting

Here's what nobody tells you: every skipped day trains your brain.

Every time you say, "I'll start tomorrow," you're wiring your mind to believe your excuses win.

You're teaching yourself that your word means nothing.

And once you've reinforced that pattern enough times, quitting becomes your identity.

That's why showing up matters. It's not about the calories burned or the weight lifted. It's about proving to yourself that you can be trusted.

My Hardest Days

There were days I had migraines so bad it felt like a drill was going through my skull. I'd lie in the dark and think, Not today. I can't.

But then I'd remind myself: life isn't asking if I'm ready. Life is already here.

There were mornings after back-to-back shifts where my knees were swollen, my lungs burned from sleep apnea, and just putting on my shoes felt like war.

But I knew if I didn't show up today, I wouldn't show up tomorrow. And if I didn't show up tomorrow, I might never show up again.

I had days where my depression whispered, Disappear. Nobody will care.

But then I remembered the shake after the doctor's words, and how that shake didn't save me. It only buried me.

So I made a rule: even if I only had 1% left, I would give that 1%.

The Power of 1%

Progress doesn't come from giant leaps. It comes from stacking small wins.

- ▶ One walk instead of skipping the gym.
- ▶ One clean meal instead of fast food.
- ▶ One liter of water instead of soda.

That 1% proof stacks higher than any "all-or-nothing" crash diet ever will.

And here's the truth: 1% on a bad day is more powerful than 100% on a good day.

Because 1% on a bad day proves your discipline is real.

The Identity Shift

I stopped waiting to feel ready. I stopped waiting for motivation.

Instead, I became the man who shows up regardless.

Not "fit guy." Not "motivated guy." Not "perfect diet guy."

Just the man who shows up.

That identity is unbreakable.

The Navy Lesson

In the Navy, showing up wasn't optional. The mission didn't wait because you were tired. The team didn't stop because you had excuses.

You showed up, or you let everyone down.

And that's the same mindset I carried into weight loss.

Every workout was a mission. Every meal was a mission. Every step was a mission.

It wasn't about liking it. It was about executing it.

Excuses Are Comfort in Disguise

- Pain gives you an excuse.
- Fatigue gives you an excuse.
- Cravings give you an excuse.
- Stress gives you an excuse.

But excuses don't care if you live or die. Excuses don't care about your kids, your spouse, or your future.

Excuses are comfort in disguise. And comfort is the slowest poison in the world.

A Story of a 1% Day

There was a morning I'd only slept two hours. My body was wrecked. My brain foggy.

Everything in me said, No way today.

But my rule was simple: I show up no matter what.

So I laced my shoes. Walked outside. Didn't sprint. Didn't break records. I just walked.

By the end of that walk, I wasn't proud of the distance. I was proud of the proof.

Because I showed up. And that's all it took to keep momentum alive.

The Compound Effect

Here's what happens when you show up, even on the days you don't want to:

- You build trust with yourself.
- You kill the cycle of excuses.
- You prove discipline > motivation.
- You keep momentum alive.

And those ugly, tired, broken days? They become the victories you remember most.

The workouts I remember aren't the ones where I crushed it. They're the ones where I didn't want to be there—but I was.

Tactical Weapons to Win the Day

Here are the tools I used to win the days I didn't want to show up:

▶ **The 5-Minute Rule:** Commit to five minutes. If you still want to quit after, you can. (You won't.)

▶ **The Countdown Rule:** 5–4–3–2–1. Move. Don't think.

▶ **The Anchor Rule:** "I'm the kind of person who shows up no matter what." Identity > excuses.

▶ **The Lay It Out Rule:** Shoes by the door. Clothes ready. Remove excuses before they whisper.

▶ **The Micro-Proof Rule:** Stack one undeniable proof every day. Water. Steps. Meal. Doesn't matter, proof stacks.

What's Really at Stake

Let me be blunt: every time you don't show up, you're gambling with your life.

▶ That skipped workout? It's not just a workout. It's momentum lost.

▶ That late-night binge? It's not just calories. It's proof you let weakness win.

▶ That excuse? It's not just today. It's your identity on the line.

When you don't show up, you're not just pausing your progress. You're voting for the old you to live longer.

The Curveball Connection

Life will always throw curveballs.
The question isn't whether the pitch is fair. The question is whether you swing anyway.

I've been hit with curveballs that knocked me flat: pink slips, repos, depression, nearly 400 pounds of weight crushing my chest.

But every curveball forced me to make a choice: freeze, or swing.
And every time I swung. No matter how ugly the swing, it kept me alive.
That's what showing up is. Swinging ugly, but swinging anyway.

Your Move

So here's your battle plan:

Stop waiting for motivation.
Stop waiting for perfect conditions.
Stop waiting until you "feel like it."

Show up anyway.

Even broken. Even tired. Even afraid. Even doubtful.

Because the person who shows up when they don't want to is the one who wins in the end.

Final Word

At 21, nearly 400 pounds, the doctors said I wouldn't make it past 23.

And the first thing I did? I didn't show up. I bought a shake.

But that shake didn't save me. It buried me.

The only thing that ever saved me was showing up—again and again and again.

So when the day comes that you don't want to show up, remember: that day matters most.

Not showing up doesn't erase the problem. Facing it does.
So face it. Conquer it. Repeat.
Because the days you don't want to show up are the days that decide your future.

CHAPTER 17

Environment Is Everything

Change Your Surroundings, Change Your Life

Set up your environment for your worst day, not your best because that day decides your success. Weight loss isn't about willpower, it's about preparing for weakness, not strength.

The Kitchen That Attacked Me

When I tell people that environment is everything, they nod. They think they get it. "Yeah, Cristian, don't keep junk food in the house. I get it."

No. You don't get it. Not until you've been where I was.

Sabotage isn't just about willpower when you're awake. It's deeper than that. Sabotage can live in your environment so strongly it reaches into your subconscious. It hunts you when you're weakest.

I wasn't a late-night snacker. That's cute. That's innocent. I was a night eater.

I would literally break my own sleep, stumble to the fridge like a drunk, and inhale food half-asleep—not because I was hungry, not because I chose to, but because my environment had written the script hours earlier.

The Night I Woke Up Inside the Fridge

It was 2 a.m.

Maybe 3.

I don't remember the exact time, because I wasn't awake. Not fully. My mind was fogged, but my body was moving.

I stumbled through the house like a drunk zombie, eyes half-closed, lungs barely breathing through sleep apnea, feet heavy on the tile. And without a single conscious thought, I went straight to the kitchen. Straight to the fridge.

The door thumped open. Cold air hit my face. And I went in.
I went in fast. Real fast.
Not for water. Not for anything I actually needed.
For cookies.

M&M cookies. A whole pack sat there waiting. I tore them open without a thought, shoving one after another into my mouth, barely chewing, barely tasting. I wasn't eating because I was hungry. I wasn't even tasting them. I was eating because they were there.

And cookies need something to wash them down, right? That reflex was still alive even half-asleep. I grabbed the carton in the door and started chugging.

Only it wasn't milk.
It was raw egg whites.

By the time my wife rushed in, woken by the commotion; half my body was inside the refrigerator, cookie crumbs down my shirt, an empty egg-white carton dangling from my hand like a trophy.

She stared at me in shock. I stared back in shame, but I wasn't fully there. I was asleep with my eyes open. My body had taken over.

That's how powerful environment is. That's what sabotage looks like. I was eating before tasting. Eating without knowing.

And in that moment I realized something terrifying: my environment was stronger than my consciousness.

The Psychology of Night Eating

Here's what science confirms:

▸ Your brain doesn't "forget" food. If it's in your environment, your subconscious remembers exactly where it is.

▸ Memory + reward loops. Eat cookies once from a certain place and your brain records the location, the smell, the feeling. Next time, it doesn't "ask" you. It drags you back.

▸ Circadian sabotage. At night, hunger hormones like ghrelin can spike and fullness signals like leptin can dip. Your decision-making (prefrontal cortex) is tired while your emotional drives (amygdala) stay active. Translation: logic is asleep, cravings are awake.

▸ Environment is the trigger. If there were no cookies in the fridge, there would've been no 2 a.m. massacre.

It wasn't that I was weak. My environment was designed for me to lose.

The Fix: Starve the House

After that night, I knew something had to change.
I didn't need more willpower. I needed an advantage.
I stripped my environment bare:

▸ Rule #1: If it tempts you at 2 a.m., it doesn't belong in your house at 2 p.m.

▸ Rule #2: Visibility = vulnerability. Anything in eyesight becomes a guaranteed craving. Out of sight isn't out of mind, but it's one less bullet fired at you.

▶ Rule #3: Flood the kitchen with proof. Replace sabotage foods with mission food. If I raided the fridge half-asleep, at least the raid would help me win.

And it worked. Sometimes I still woke up. I still shuffled to the kitchen. But instead of inhaling M&M cookies with raw egg whites, I grabbed water or a piece of lean protein. The environment shifted from sabotage to support.

Why This Matters to You

If you're struggling, stop blaming willpower. Stop calling yourself "undisciplined." You're not failing because you're weak. You're failing because your environment is built for sabotage.

Think about it:

▶ Why do you always want chips at night?
▶ Why do you "accidentally" grab cookies with your coffee?
▶ Why does every diet collapse around 9 p.m.?

It's not that you don't want it bad enough. It's that you're walking into a battlefield where every weapon is pointed at you.

Your Mission: The Midnight Audit

Tonight, run a simple mission, the Midnight Audit.

When the house is quiet, walk into your kitchen and look around. Be brutally honest.

Ask yourself:

▶ If I woke up half-asleep right now, what would I grab first?
▶ If my weakest self raided this fridge, would it help me win, or guarantee I lose?

That answer is your proof. That's your environment exposing you.

Now clean house. Not tomorrow. Not next week. Now. Strip it bare. Flood it with proof. If your weakest version can still win in that kitchen, your strongest version becomes unstoppable.

Eating Without Tasting
That night wasn't unique. I did it often.
Not eating because I was hungry. Eating because food existed within reach.

Sometimes it was cookies.
Sometimes cereal.
Sometimes spoonfuls of peanut butter straight from the jar.

I didn't even taste it. It wasn't pleasure, it was compulsion. My environment was set up for failure, and I was just following the script.

Food should be fuel. I was using it like a drug, swallowing calories without thought, taste, or awareness.

If you've ever stood in the kitchen at night, staring into the light of the fridge, eating something you didn't even want, you know exactly what I'm talking about.

That isn't personal failure. That's engineered failure.

Why Environment Beats Willpower

People talk about willpower like it's a magic muscle—"Just try harder."

It doesn't work like that.

Willpower drains. When you're tired, stressed, or emotionally fried, it vanishes. That's why your house has to be a fortress.

Environment beats willpower every time:

- If the cookies aren't in the fridge, you can't eat them at 2 a.m.
- If the soda isn't in the pantry, you can't crack it after a bad day.

> ▶ If the chips aren't in your car, you can't snack on them while driving.

The body can't eat what isn't there.

That night I raided the fridge, it wasn't about discipline. It was about design. I had built a kitchen that was set up to kill me. And it almost did.

The Kitchen That Kills You

Look at your kitchen right now. Is it proof or sabotage?

> ▶ Fridge: What's the first thing you see, soda, leftover pizza, or clean protein?
> ▶ Pantry: Chips, cookies, crackers—or rice, oats, canned tuna?
> ▶ Freezer: Ice cream and frozen dinners—or chicken, vegetables, frozen fruit?

Every item is a weapon. Every shelf is a decision waiting to happen.

That night at 2 a.m., my fridge was loaded like an enemy arsenal. My subconscious knew it. That's why it dragged me there half-asleep.

If you want to win this war, strip the enemy of its weapons.

The Fridge Purge

The single most powerful thing I did wasn't cardio. It wasn't lifting. It wasn't fasting.

It was purging my kitchen.

I threw away every sabotage food.

Not "save it for the kids."
Not "for guests."
Not "just in case."

Gone.

If it wasn't proof, it didn't make the cut.

Was it easy? No. I felt wasteful. Guilty. Like I was throwing money away. But here's what I learned: every cookie I tossed was a heart attack I dodged. Every soda I dumped was a step toward being alive for my kids.

That purge saved my life.

Proof Foods: Build a Fortress

After the purge, I didn't leave emptiness. I rebuilt with proof:

- ▶ Chicken tenderloins
- ▶ Lean beef (96/4)
- ▶ Eggs
- ▶ Plain Greek yogurt
- ▶ Rice
- ▶ Spinach
- ▶ Avocado (yes, even if you hate it, a little daily stacks up)
- ▶ Fruit (apples, berries, bananas)

My fridge became an ally. My pantry became an ammo crate. My freezer became a fallback.

The first time I half-slept my way to the kitchen after that? I opened the door, reached in blind, grabbed Greek yogurt, ate it, and went back to bed.

That's the power of environment: when you're at your weakest, it decides whether you win or lose.

How to Beat the 2 A.M. Enemy (Tactics)

1) The Midnight Audit Drill

Before bed tonight, walk your kitchen like a burglar. Open every cabinet, fridge, freezer, and drawer. Ask: If I woke up half-asleep right now, what would I grab? If the answer isn't something you're proud of, it's got to go.

2) The Visibility Rule

If it's visible, it's vulnerable. No chips on the counter. No soda in plain sight. No candy bowls "for guests."

3) The Sabotage Detox

Throw it out. All of it. If it's not proof, it's poison. You're not wasting food. You're saving your life.

4) The Proof Swap List

- ▶ Cookies → Greek yogurt + berries
- ▶ Chips → air-popped popcorn
- ▶ Soda → sparkling water + lime
- ▶ Ice cream → frozen banana blended with protein

5) The 2 A.M. Plan

Keep two "emergency wins" in the fridge at all times:

- ▶ a measured portion of lean protein (ready-to-eat), and
- ▶ a bottle of cold water front-row center.

If you raid half-asleep, you still win.

6) The Layout Advantage

Put water and protein at eye level. Push "sometimes foods" (even the clean ones) to lower shelves. Your eyes choose before your brain does.

Mindset Flip: You're Not Weak. Your Kitchen Was.

Listen. This matters.

You're not weak because you've raided the fridge at night. You're not broken because you've eaten half-asleep.

You're human. And your environment was engineered to beat you.

Weakness isn't permanent. Environment isn't fixed. You can strip the triggers. You can re-arm your kitchen with proof. You can win even at your weakest.

Your Opportunity

Here's your challenge:

- ▸ Purge your kitchen this week.
- ▸ Restock with proof.
- ▸ Run the Midnight Audit and feel the difference when you open a fridge that has your back instead of its hands around your throat.

Because here's the truth:

Discipline doesn't live in your head 24/7.
It lives in your kitchen.

Time to Lock in

The 2 a.m. enemy isn't hunger. It isn't weakness. It isn't even you.
It's sabotage, and sabotage only wins if you let it.

The night I inhaled cookies and raw egg whites, I wasn't broken. I was unarmed. My kitchen had been turned against me.

Once I rebuilt it, the war changed.
Now, even if I wake up half-asleep, stumbling to the fridge, I win, because even at my weakest, my environment fights for me, not against me.

That's the key. That's the proof. That's how you win, by turning your kitchen from an enemy outpost into a stronghold.

So lock it in.
Do the purge.
Stack the proof.

Even at 2 a.m., half-asleep, you can still win if your environment is built for victory.

The Kitchen That Changed Everything

When people ask me what finally flipped the switch in my journey, they expect me to say something about willpower, motivation, or the perfect workout. But the truth is simpler, and more ruthless.

It was my kitchen.

I remember standing in the middle of it one night, staring at the wreckage of my old life. Pizza boxes stacked like sandbags. Crushed soda cans rolling under my feet. Open bags of chips spread across the counter like landmines waiting to be stepped on. It wasn't just a kitchen, it was a battlefield.

Everywhere I looked, weakness had already won.

And in that moment, it hit me: my environment was designing my choices before I ever made them. I wasn't failing because I lacked discipline. I was failing because my terrain was built for defeat.

So I cleaned house. Literally. I bagged the chips, dumped the soda, and cleared the counter. I rebuilt the kitchen the way a soldier builds a base: stocked, organized, and impossible to mistake for enemy territory. Chicken, rice, spinach, water jugs, Greek yogurt. Nothing else.

That night wasn't about food. It was about war. And the kitchen was my first fortress.

Terrain Wins Wars

Every general knows terrain matters more than tactics. You can have the best soldiers in the world, but if you're fighting uphill in mud while the enemy fires downhill, you're dead before you start.

Your environment is your terrain. If it's tilted against you, no amount of hype will save you.

Think about it:

▶ A man who drives past three fast-food restaurants on the way home has to fight temptation three times a day.

▶ A woman who keeps cookies "for the kids" on the counter has to win a staring contest with sugar every time she pours coffee.

▶ Someone who falls asleep with their phone in hand isn't losing sleep because they're weak. They're losing sleep because their environment is wired to rob them.

You don't beat that with motivation. You beat it by changing the ground you stand on.

The Four Environments

There are four environments you must master:

1. Physical – the spaces you live, eat, sleep, and train in.
2. Digital – the devices, apps, and screens that dictate your focus.
3. Mental – the internal landscape of stories you tell yourself.
4. Social – the people, cultures, and communities you allow around you.

Ignore one, and it will sabotage you. Master all four, and you become untouchable.

1. The Physical Environment

Your house, your car, your workspace, they're either allies or enemies.

When I was at my heaviest, my physical environment was an ambush waiting to happen. Vending machines at work. Gas station snacks during commutes. A pantry that looked like a junk food warehouse.

I realized I couldn't keep walking into traps and expect to walk out victorious. So I rebuilt.

Rules of the Physical Battlefield:

▸ Starve the house. If it's not in the house, it can't attack you. Your pantry is either proof or poison.

▸ Flood it with proof. Water jugs on the counter. Chicken thawing in the fridge. Protein ready to cook. Make success the default.

▸ Design choke points. Put your workout shoes by the door. Keep a pull-up bar in the hallway. Force your environment to push you toward action.

Every pound I lost started in my physical environment. Because when your terrain supports your mission, discipline feels effortless.

2. The Digital Environment

Your phone is a weapon, or a landmine.

Scroll long enough, and you'll find endless food porn, fake experts, and dopamine traps engineered to hijack your brain. And here's the truth: willpower doesn't beat algorithms. You have to rewire your digital battlefield.

Tactics for the Digital War:

▸ App purge. Delete the apps that pull you off mission. Every swipe is either proof stacked or proof stolen.

- Kill notifications. Every buzz is an ambush. Silence them. Control when you engage.
- Follow proof only. If your feed doesn't inspire action, it's sabotaging you. Fill it with fitness, discipline, and people living the life you want.

When I rebuilt my digital environment, I stopped waking up to chaos and started waking up to proof. My phone went from enemy agent to battle ally.

3. The Mental Environment

This is the hardest terrain of all, your own head.

When I was 370 pounds, my mental environment was a swamp of excuses. "I'll start Monday." "One soda won't hurt." "My genetics are bad." Every thought was quicksand pulling me under.

The breakthrough came when I realized I could re-engineer my mental terrain the same way I rebuilt my kitchen. Every negative thought had to be starved out and replaced with proof.

Rebuilding the Mental Environment:

- Audit your thoughts. Write down the three excuses you tell yourself most often. That's your enemy playbook. Burn it.
- Replace with proof. For every excuse, stack evidence. "I can't run" becomes "I ran mailbox to mailbox yesterday."
- Guard the gates. Don't let weakness rent space in your head. Thoughts are squatters, you evict them by moving, not debating.

Your mental environment is the command center. If it's compromised, the mission fails. Guard it like a fortress.

4. The Social Environment

Show me your circle, I'll show you your future.

I didn't understand this at first. I thought I could drag my old crowd with me into my new life. But the truth is, some people would rather see you stay stuck so they don't feel left behind.

When I started stacking proof, the jokes rolled in. "Lighten up, bro." "One bite won't kill you." "Don't get too obsessed." They weren't trying to kill me, but their words were bullets all the same.

So I built a new social environment. People who understood the mission. People who stacked proof themselves. People who pushed me forward, not pulled me back.

Rules for the Social Battlefield:

▶ Identify anchors. Who drags you back to old habits? Cut the rope.
▶ Find allies. Even one battle buddy doubles your strength.
▶ Lead from the front. Your discipline will inspire more than your words ever will.

Your environment isn't just walls and screens. It's people. And if those people don't serve your mission, they serve your destruction.

Routine: The Operating System

Environment builds the terrain. But routine? That's the operating system.

Without routine, your environment is just a room full of objects. With routine, it's a fortress.

Every morning, my routine was the same: wake up, hydrate, move, eat protein. It wasn't glamorous. It wasn't exciting. But it was bulletproof.

Why? Because routine kills negotiation. When you live by routine, you don't waste energy deciding whether or not to act. You just act.

Think of a pilot before takeoff. Every switch, every dial, every lever checked in the same order every time. That routine saves lives. Yours can too.

Missions for the Reader

1. Kitchen Reset Mission – Tonight, clear your kitchen of everything that doesn't serve your mission. Replace it with lean protein, vegetables, and water.
2. Phone Rebuild Mission – Delete three apps that drain you. Follow three people who push you forward.
3. Mental Audit Mission – Write down your three biggest excuses. Replace each with one proof you've stacked this week.
4. Social Checkpoint Mission – Identify one anchor relationship. Have the hard conversation, or create space.

Lock It In

Environment isn't decoration. It's destiny.

You don't rise to the level of your goals, you fall to the level of your environment.

When you walk into a kitchen designed for proof, you win before you start.

When your phone feeds you discipline instead of dopamine, you win before you swipe.

When your thoughts are fortified and your circle pushes you forward, you win before you fight.

That's why environment is everything.

Because in the end, success isn't built on hype. It's built on proof. And proof is stacked one choice at a time, in the environment you control.

CHAPTER 18

This Is Not a Diet

Everywhere you turn, there's a new "plan."

Keto. Paleo. Vegan. Carnivore. Intermittent fasting. Low-fat. Low-carb. Juice cleanses.

Each one promises transformation. Each one hooks you with hype. And each one has the same problem: they're diets.

Diets end. Diets yo-yo. Diets give you an exit strategy back to weakness.

What I built isn't a diet.
It's a system.
The CL System.

A war plan with no gray areas, no excuses, no leeway.

You don't negotiate with cravings.
You don't debate with weakness.
You don't "try" to follow rules.
You execute. Every day. Even when you don't feel like it.

Because this isn't keto. This isn't paleo.

This is war.

The Problem With Diets

Here's the hard truth:

> ▶ Keto works — until the first slice of bread.
> ▶ Paleo works — until the first pizza.

▶ Vegan works — until the cheese cravings hit.

▶ Intermittent fasting works — until the late-night snack sneaks in.

Every diet gives you a window back to your old self.
And the old self always takes it.

That's why people yo-yo. They drop 20, gain 30. They drop 50, gain 60.
They live their lives in cycles of hype and collapse.
Diets change your food. They don't change you.

The CL System changes both.

The CL System: No Gray Areas

I built this system out of necessity. At 370+ pounds, I didn't need another plan. I needed a battlefield manual.

The rules were clear.

▶ Protein is non-negotiable.

▶ Grams don't lie.

▶ Steps equal sanity.

▶ Sleep debt equals snack debt.

▶ Move to kill the urge.

▶ Starve the traps.

▶ Proof over plateaus.

▶ The new you is non-negotiable.

This isn't about switching one food for another. It's about eliminating weakness entirely. Cutting it off at the root.

You don't get to live in the gray. Gray is where excuses breed. Gray is where diets fail.

With the CL System, it's black or white. You're in or you're out. You stack proof or you stack excuses.

Why This Lasts

The reason diets fail is because they're temporary identities. "I'm keto for 30 days." "I'm fasting this week." "I'm doing Whole30."

When the clock runs out, so does the discipline.

The CL System lasts because it isn't a program, it's a transformation. It's permanent. Once you bury the old you, there's no going back.

You don't "try keto." You become disciplined.
You don't "test intermittent fasting." You become proof-stacking.
You don't "go paleo." You become ruthless.

That's why this system works for life.

The Difference in the Field

Imagine two soldiers.

One is following a "diet." His ammo is limited. His strategy is borrowed. He fights as long as the weather holds. The first obstacle, he runs out of gas.

The other follows the CL System. His ammo is discipline. His strategy is identity. He fights no matter the terrain, no matter the obstacle. He adapts, adjusts, attacks. And he wins.

That's the difference between keto and this system. Between diet and discipline.

Real World Tactics

Here's what makes the CL System different:

- No cheat meals. You don't reward discipline by feeding weakness.
- Superfoods stacked daily. Even if you hate them. Small doses that add up. (Remember avocado.)

- ▶ Grams over guesses. You measure every bite. No "close enough." No "eyeballing."
- ▶ Fallback rules. On the road? Traveling? The only fallback is whole protein. Not fast food, not candy bars, not "just this once."
- ▶ Environment wins. Weakness can't tempt you if it's not in your house. That's why you starve the traps.
- ▶ MTKU (Move to Kill the Urge). Craving? You move. Urge gone. Simple, effective, undefeated.

These aren't suggestions. They're laws. Break them and you break yourself. Follow them and you transform.

The Mental Shift

You want lasting change?
Stop calling it a diet. Stop treating it like an experiment. Stop making it seasonal.

This is not keto. This is not paleo. This is not Atkins. This is not vegan. This is war.
And in war, you don't play games.

The battlefield is your body. The enemy is weakness. The CL System is your weapon.

No yo-yo. No gray area. No going back.

Your Move

- ▶ Stop looking for diets. Start living discipline.
- ▶ Stop negotiating with cravings. Start eliminating them.
- ▶ Stop stacking excuses. Start stacking proof.

This is the A–Z route. No detours. No rest stops. No "I'll get back on track Monday."

You march until the war is won.

Lock It In

The CL System isn't a diet. It's the end of diets.

Because this isn't about food swaps. This is about identity swaps. The old you is dead. The new you is permanent.

This is not keto. This is not a diet. This is war.

The CL System Creed

This is not keto.
This is not a diet.

This is war. And the fight is your freedom. The freedom to take your shirt off comfortably again, the freedom to go to a restaurant once in a while with friends and choose whatever, the freedom to find yourself again

I don't negotiate with cravings.
I don't debate with weakness.
I don't wait for motivation.
I move, I fight, I finish.

I measure every gram.
I stack every proof.
I starve every trap.
I protect my sleep.
I guard my foxhole.

The old me is dead.
The new me is permanent.
The new me is non-negotiable.

And my motto is simple:

"The workout doesn't stop until you do."

CHAPTER 19

The New You Is Non-Negotiable

The old you died the day you declared war.

The weak version. The excuse-maker. The binge-eater. The man who hid from the mirror.

You buried him with every step, every gram, every mile, every night you strapped in and fought through cravings.

Now you stand here, proof stacked higher than doubt, and the only rule left is this:

The new you is non-negotiable.

The Illusion of "Going Back"

Most people lose weight or make progress only to relapse. Why? Because they see discipline as temporary. A diet. A program. A challenge. Something with an end date.

That's why they go back.

But the truth is simple: **there is no going back.** Once you've crossed the battlefield, once you've proven what's possible, once you've tasted strength, going back is death.

The new you isn't a season. It's a soldier. Permanent. Non-negotiable.

Identity Over Options

Weakness thrives in options. "Maybe I'll run today." "Maybe I'll weigh my food." "Maybe I'll get back on track Monday."

Options are exits, and exits lead back to the old you.

The new you removes exits. Discipline isn't a choice anymore. It's identity.

- ▸ You don't try to hit your steps. You hit them.
- ▸ You don't consider your fast. You hold the line.
- ▸ You don't debate protein. You eat it.
- ▸ You don't negotiate with traps. You starve them.

The new you doesn't choose. The new you commands.

Proof Beyond the Scale

By now you've learned: plateaus are illusions, sleep debt is snack debt, grams don't lie, and steps equal sanity. You've proven yourself in the trenches.

The new you doesn't live by the scale.
The new you lives by proof.

Every step tracked, every urge killed, every night of sleep protected, these are your medals of honor.

The old you measured life by pounds.
The new you measures life by proof.

Non-Negotiables = Freedom

People think non-negotiables are restrictions. They're not. They're freedom.

Freedom from guilt.
Freedom from bargaining with weakness.
Freedom from the loop of starting over again and again.

When the rules are non-negotiable, there's no decision fatigue. You know exactly what to do, every day, no matter what battlefield you wake up on.

Non-negotiables simplify life. They cut through chaos. They guarantee results.

The War Story

When I was 400+ pounds, I lived in negotiation. I negotiated with the snooze button. I negotiated with fast food. I negotiated with soda. Every negotiation ended the same: I lost.

When I went all-in, when I declared war, I removed the negotiation table. Weakness had no vote. Cravings had no microphone. Excuses had no chair.

That's when I became dangerous. That's when the old me died and the new me became permanent.

Building Your Non-Negotiables

Here's how you lock it down:

1. **Steps:** 10k+ a day. No excuses. Rain, snow, heat — steps stack regardless.
2. **Protein:** 1–2 grams per pound of goal weight. Every day. No skipping.
3. **Grams:** Food measured. Not eyeballed. Not "close enough." Logged in proof.
4. **Fasting:** Daily window. Minimum 14 hours. Kitchen closed at curfew.
5. **Sleep:** 7–8 hours, CPAP strapped, curfew respected.
6. **Environment:** Starve the traps. If it's poison, it doesn't enter your house.
7. **MTKU:** Move to kill urges. Immediate. Non-negotiable.
8. **Mindset:** Proof over plateaus. Progress over excuses. Always.

If you lock these eight rules into identity, there's no negotiation left. You don't decide daily. You execute daily.

Example: The Firefighter Rule

Think of a firefighter. When the alarm goes off, he doesn't debate whether to respond. He doesn't check his mood or motivation. His identity is firefighter. He moves without question.

That's how the new you operates. Alarm goes off —> you move. Fast window closes —> you stop. Steps unfinished —> you walk. Craving hits —> you kill it.

It's not debate. It's discipline.

The Enemy Always Knocks

Don't get it twisted, weakness doesn't disappear. It knocks on the door daily.

The old you opened the door and invited it in.

The new you keeps the door locked.

Weakness Doesn't Just Knock, It Sneaks

Weakness isn't always loud. Sometimes it doesn't come banging on the door, it sneaks through the cracks.

It waits for your weakest moments.

- ▶ When you're exhausted after a 12 hour shift.
- ▶ When you're fighting with your spouse.
- ▶ When you've been clean for weeks and your guard drops for one second.

That's when it whispers:

"Just one bite."
"Just this once."
"You've earned it."

And before you know it, one compromise turns into a chain reaction.

That's why the new you is non-negotiable. Because weakness doesn't demand all of you at once, it takes inches. It chips away until you're right back where you started.

I remember one night, months into my war, standing in front of a gas station cooler at midnight. I wasn't even hungry. I was tired. Angry. Frustrated. And there it was, rows of soda, the old poison calling me back. For two minutes, I actually convinced myself I "deserved" it.

That was weakness attacking me in silence, not noise.
But I walked out empty-handed. That was traction over temptation.
Weakness doesn't storm the gates. It sneaks in through the cracks.

That's why you seal the cracks. That's why the new you is non-negotiable.

The old you opened the door and invited it in.

The new you keeps the door locked.

Every day, weakness knocks. Every day, the new you refuses to answer.

Field Test

From this chapter forward, your life is non-negotiable discipline. The new you isn't optional. It isn't seasonal. It isn't fragile.

- ▸ No debating with weakness.
- ▸ No bargaining with cravings.
- ▸ No exits, no detours, no "later."
- ▸ Proof stacked daily until the mission is complete.

This isn't about willpower. It's about identity. The old you is dead. The new you is permanent.

Non-Negotiable

The old you negotiated. The old you lost. The old you lived in chains.

The new you commands. The new you wins. The new you is free.

The new you is non-negotiable.

CHAPTER 20
Survival to Significance

The Trap of Survival

Life doesn't begin with freedom. It begins with survival.

I know what it feels like to wake up already tired. To roll over in bed with your heart racing before the day even starts. To stare at bills stacked on the counter, your stomach knotted before you even eat. To look at yourself in the mirror and see not possibility, but punishment.

That's survival mode.

For me, survival was almost 400 pounds strapped to my body. Every step felt like punishment. My chest heaved at night while sleep apnea strangled me. My blood pressure was through the roof. Doctors told me I wouldn't make it to 23.

That's not living. That's waiting to die.

And the scariest part about survival mode is this: it convinces you that "barely hanging on" is enough. That existing counts as life. That being "not dead yet" is the same as thriving.

But survival is a trap.

It blinds you to your potential. It teaches you to make decisions in 10-minute windows, not 10-year visions. It locks you into chaos, fear, and excuses until you forget what freedom even feels like.

And if you stay there too long, your biology will trap you there permanently.

Because when you live in survival mode, your nervous system sits in fight-or-flight every single day. Cortisol runs wild. Your body thinks you're being hunted. And when your body thinks you're prey, you don't dream about building. You just pray about surviving.

I know this truth because I lived it. I lived stuck in survival for years. But survival isn't permanent.

There's a ladder out.

The Traction Code

That ladder is what I call The Traction Code.
It's not a diet. It's not a trend. It's not a motivational quote you slap on your wall.

It's a framework, one that I had to discover the hard way, through failure, through pain, through setbacks that nearly broke me.

There are five stages in the Traction Code:

1. Survival – Barely hanging on. Reactive. Drowning in chaos.
2. Stability – Creating a foundation. Routine. Order. Breathing room.
3. Strength – Building power. Identity shift. Confidence.
4. Significance – Living for something bigger than yourself.
5. Service – Legacy. Impact. Proof that outlives you.

Every human lives somewhere on this ladder. Some stay stuck on the bottom rung until the day they die. Some climb, then slip back down. But a rare few climb all the way, and those are the ones who change their lives and the lives around them.

That's what I want for you.

The beauty of this code is that it doesn't lie. It doesn't flatter. It doesn't sugarcoat. It shows you exactly where you are, and exactly what you need to do next.

Stage One – Survival

Survival looks like this:

- You live paycheck to paycheck.
- You eat whatever numbs the pain, not what fuels your body.
- You wake up tired, go to bed tired, and live tired in between.
- You put out fires all day but never build anything permanent.
- Every decision is about the next craving, the next bill, the next escape.

In survival, the smallest problem feels like the end of the world. A flat tire isn't an inconvenience, it's a catastrophe. A bad day at work feels like proof your whole life is collapsing.

And in survival, you become addicted to the wrong questions:

- "Why me?"
- "How do I get through this day?"
- "What's the fastest way to escape this feeling?"

The biology matches the psychology. Survival is cortisol. Survival is shallow breathing. Survival is tunnel vision.

The tragedy of survival is that it doesn't just rob you of joy. It robs you of imagination. When your nervous system is locked in fight-or-flight, you can't see beyond the lion chasing you.

And if you don't see the ladder, you can't climb it.

Stage Two – Stability

Stability is where you take your first step out of the pit.

It doesn't mean life is perfect. It doesn't mean all your problems disappear. It means you finally stop living in chaos long enough to breathe.

Stability looks like this:

- You create a daily routine.
- You meal prep instead of winging it.
- You schedule your workouts instead of hoping for time.
- You budget your money instead of letting it slip through your fingers.

Stability is built on rhythm, not randomness.

When I was in survival mode, my life had no rhythm. I ate whatever was around. Slept whenever I crashed. Worked when I was forced to. Chaos was my soundtrack.

But when I locked in routines, meals, workouts, sleep my nervous system calmed. My body shifted out of panic. My mind could finally focus.

That's the gift of stability: it trades chaos for clarity.

People in survival say, "I don't have time." People in stability say, "This is my time."

And that's the difference.

Stage Three – Strength

Once stability is locked, you can build strength.

Strength isn't just biceps and squats. Strength is identity. It's the moment you stop saying, "I'm trying to lose weight" and start saying, "I'm disciplined."

Strength is proof stacked. Every time you make a promise and keep it, you become someone new. Every rep in the gym, every meal logged, every bill paid on time, brick by brick you build a fortress of identity.

When I moved into strength, something shifted. People around me felt it. I wasn't "trying" anymore. I was becoming.

Strength is contagious. Your spouse feels it. Your kids see it. Your coworkers notice it.

Because strength isn't about what you say. It's about what you are.

Stage Four – Significance

Significance is when the mission expands beyond you.

It's not just about losing 50 pounds or paying off debt. It's about purpose.

Significance is when your kids see you as a leader. When your spouse feels secure in your presence. When your transformation lights a path for someone else.

This is where science confirms what spirituality always knew: dopamine rewards you for winning alone, but serotonin rewards you for lifting others.

Serotonin is the chemistry of respect, belonging, leadership. It's what makes you stand taller, speak stronger, live bolder.

When you hit significance, life stops being about ego. It becomes about mission.

Stage Five – Service

The highest rung is service.

This is where you stop asking, "What do I get?" and start asking, "What do I give?"

Service is building a legacy. Service is proof that outlives you.

When I host Traction Retreats, when I coach one-on-one, when I write these words, I'm in service. Not because I want applause, but because I refuse to let my proof die with me.

And here's what science shows: people who live in service live longer, healthier, happier lives. Stress decreases. Meaning increases. Health improves.

Service is where survival turns to immortality.

The Ladder of Traction

Picture a ladder.

- Bottom rung: Survival.
- Middle rungs: Stability and Strength.
- Top rungs: Significance and Service.

You can't skip rungs. You can't leap from survival to significance. But you can climb one at a time.
The code is simple:

- Survival → Stability: Replace chaos with rhythm.
- Stability → Strength: Replace excuses with proof.
- Strength → Significance: Replace ego with purpose.
- Significance → Service: Replace self with legacy.

That's the Traction Code.

The Cost of Staying Stuck

Let's get blunt.
If you stay in survival:

- Your health will collapse.
- Your relationships will wither.
- Your potential will rot inside you until the day you die.

And the only thing you'll leave behind are excuses, regrets, and what-ifs.

That's the cost of staying stuck.

But if you climb, if you embrace the Traction Code, the cost flips. You'll pay in discipline, but the reward will be freedom.

Daily Proof – The Code in Action

Here's how to climb daily:

- ▶ Journal: clarity.
- ▶ Breath work: calm.
- ▶ Training: resilience.
- ▶ Nutrition: fuel.
- ▶ Service: fulfillment.

You don't have to master all five stages at once. Just master the rung you're on.

That's the genius of the code: it meets you exactly where you are.

Reader Challenges

1. Survival Check: Write down where you're surviving. Money? Food? Sleep? Relationships? Name it. That's your battlefield.
2. Stability Ritual: Pick one boring, consistent action you'll do daily for the next 7 days. Same time, same way. Prove rhythm.
3. Strength Stack: Choose one promise you'll keep every day this week. Track it. Build bricks.
4. Significance Shift: Serve someone else daily. Small or big. Watch how it changes your energy.
5. Service Vision: Write down the legacy you want your kids or community to see when you're gone. Let that vision pull you.

Lock It In

Here's the truth:

Life doesn't reward survival. It rewards traction.

The grind doesn't matter if it doesn't move you forward. Chaos doesn't make you strong, rhythm does. Ego doesn't make you great, purpose does.

The Traction Code isn't a theory. It's proof. Proof that anyone from 400 pounds and hopeless to lean, focused, and free can climb.

Now it's your move.

Stop surviving. Start climbing.

Because the world doesn't need another spectator.

It needs proof.

And that proof is you.

CHAPTER 21

The Prospect of War

You've made it this far. You've turned the pages, underlined the lines, maybe even whispered some of them back to yourself. And deep down, something has already shifted. You don't read a war manual like this and walk away the same.

But I need to hit you with the truth.
Reading this book won't change your life.

Execution will.

The world doesn't give a damn about what you know. It only bends for what you do. You can read every diet book, every self-help manual, every blog post about motivation, but until you put steel in your spine and boots on the ground, nothing changes.

That's why I didn't write this for information. I wrote it for transformation. This isn't a cookbook. It's not a collection of tips. It's a weapon. And weapons are worthless unless you pick them up and fire.

This is your battlefield manual.
And the battlefield is your daily life.

The Prospect of the New You

Let's be clear: the old you is still lurking. The one who ate until stuffed, told lies to the mirror, promised "tomorrow," and lived in a body that felt like a prison. That man is still inside you hungry, lazy, undisciplined.

And he's waiting for you to let your guard down.

But on the other side of that enemy is the new you. The man who stacks proof every day. The man who weighs every gram, who doesn't give weakness a vote, who doesn't wait for motivation, who moves to kill the urge. The man who doesn't dabble in diets, but wages war for identity.

You've seen glimpses of him. You've felt his fire. And the prospect of living as that man isn't a fantasy, it's a decision.

But here's the truth: this system doesn't whisper. It doesn't wait. It demands.

You don't get to live in the gray. You don't get cheat meals, excuses, and "somedays."

This war doesn't have spectators. You're either in the fight or you're dead weight.

So what do you do?

You march.

Traction Retreats: The Battlefield in Real Life

That's why I created Traction Retreats. Because I know reading isn't enough. I know men need immersion. They need to feel it in their lungs, their legs, their bones.

These retreats aren't vacations. They're not spa weekends. They're military-style crucibles designed to break the old you and rebuild the new one.

What happens at a Traction Retreat?

▶ All-inclusive discipline: Every bite of food is accounted for. Every hour of sleep is protected. You're not "trying to be healthy." You're living the system.

▶ Obstacle training: We run you through dirt, water, ropes, logs, and walls. You crawl. You climb. You bleed. Because nothing carves discipline like physical adversity.

▸ Controlled discomfort: Cold plunges. Mud. Sweat. Hunger. The stuff most programs avoid, we attack head-on. Because weakness hides in comfort zones.

▸ Brotherhood: Shoulder-to-shoulder with other men in the fight. No posturing, no judgment. Just iron sharpening iron.

This isn't a "retreat." It's a Traction Retreat, the place where excuses die and the new you is born.

It's a rebirth

When you leave, your family won't just see a smaller person. They'll see a different person. A leader who shows up with strength, a partner who provides stability, a parent who inspires their kids, someone who carries themselves with fire in their eyes.

Because the retreat isn't about calories. It's about killing the old identity once and for all.

One-on-One: Traction Days

And for the men who want the fastest possible results, I built One-on-One Traction Days.

This isn't coaching calls. This isn't hand-holding. This is me, side-by-side with you, for a full day in the trenches.

We don't talk about discipline. We live it.

▸ Nutrition: You'll learn how to measure food with surgical accuracy. No eyeballing, no lies, no "close enough." You'll see how I built every meal of my journey.

▸ Movement: I'll put you through the exact same steps, reps, and miles that carried me from nearly 400 pounds down to 170. You'll hurt. You'll want to quit. And then you'll discover you have more left in the tank than you ever imagined.

▶ Treatment: Here's where it gets different. I teach you my process for preventing loose skin, accelerating fat loss, and speeding recovery.

   ○ Lymphatic drainage to flush toxins and inflammation.

   ○ Natural massage protocols that trigger circulation and skin tightening.

   ○ Systems to help your body release instead of hold on.

This is the same process I used on myself to lose 200 pounds without ending up trapped in 200 pounds of loose skin.

By the end of the day, you'll walk away not just lighter but awakened. You'll know exactly what it feels like to fight this war and win.

I tell men this straight:

These days aren't about mentorship. They're shock therapy for your life.

The Prospect of Brotherhood

Here's what makes the retreats and one-on-ones work:

▶ Knowledge without application dies.

▶ Men without brotherhood collapse.

▶ And no one climbs out of hell alone.

That's why I built this system. That's why I built these experiences. Because this isn't about motivation. It's about marching into the fire with men beside you, cadence in your ear, sweat in your eyes, and proof under your feet.

The prospect is simple:

▶ You either stay the same, trapped by weakness.

▶ Or you enter the fire and come out forged.

Weakness Attacks Slow

Before I close this war manual, you need to hear this: weakness doesn't just slam into you. It's smarter than that.

Weakness waits. It creeps. It whispers at your lowest moments, when you're tired, stressed, overwhelmed, when your guard is down. That's when it shows up with "just one bite," "just one skip," "just this once."

And if you're not ruthless, it will win.

That's why this system isn't optional. It's armor. It's weapons. It's discipline wired so deeply into your identity that when weakness comes, you're already moving, already proving, already winning.

The Final Creed

So let's end this book the only way it should end, with a creed.

Traction > Motivation.

Proof > Excuses.

The new you is non-negotiable.

I can't fight your war for you. But I can fight beside you. I can hand you the weapons. I can point to the foxhole.

The battlefield is set. The enemy is weakness. The war is yours.

And remember my motto, the one that carried me through 450 miles, 200 pounds lost, and every doubt shattered along the way:

"The workout doesn't stop until you do."

CHAPTER 22

The Recovery Key

The Lie of Endless Grind

Everyone loves the grind. Hustle culture sells it like it's holy, glorified, heroic, and divine. "No days off. Push through everything. Ignore the pain." But the truth? That mindset nearly destroyed me

And I believed it.

When I was at my heaviest, desperate to claw my way out, I thought the only answer was to push harder. More miles. More sweat. More punishment. I wore exhaustion like a badge of honor. If I collapsed at the end of a workout, I told myself I was doing it right.

But here's the truth I didn't want to face: I was lying to myself.

The grind didn't make me. It was breaking me.

Because workouts don't transform you, recovery does.

The Science Nobody Talks About

Here's the truth that almost no one explains:

- ▶ Workouts don't build muscle or burn fat. They create controlled stress. They tear you down.
- ▶ Recovery repairs the damage. That's when your body builds lean muscle, rebalances hormones, and adapts.
- ▶ Nutrition fuels the repair. Protein, carbs, fats, vitamins, minerals. Those are the building blocks of change.

- Sleep releases growth hormone. That's when tissues rebuild, inflammation drops, and fat actually burns.
- Breath, stretching, and circulation clear out lactic acid, cortisol, and stress hormones.

Workouts are the spark. Recovery is the fire.

Without recovery, your spark fizzles. Worse, it burns you out completely.

Florida, Sweat, and Puke

I'll never forget it.

Florida summer. Heat like fire pressing against my skin.

I was clocking 35 miles a week under the brutal sun. My calves were cinder blocks. My lungs rasped like sandpaper.

And almost every run ended the same way: me doubled over in the grass, puking my guts out.

At first, I thought it meant I was a warrior. "Puke means progress." That's what I told myself.

But my body was screaming a different story. Tight calves. Constant nausea. No adaptation, no progress. Just punishment.

The problem wasn't effort. The problem was recovery.

I was running on fumes. No fuel. No stretching. No structured rest. Just pain.

It wasn't until I humbled myself to the boring stuff that my body stopped revolting:

- Banana before the run. Potassium + quick carbs.
- Hydration with electrolytes. Not just water — sodium, magnesium, balance.

▶ Stretching before and after. Loosening fascia, reducing tightness.

▶ Protein after. Muscle repair on standby until you feed it.

▶ Sleep scheduled. Not "when I crash." A priority.

And you know what happened? The puking stopped. My calves loosened. My runs improved.

That lesson broke me and built me at the same time: Recovery isn't weakness. It's survival.

Why Recovery Wins the War

Let's break it down in the simplest way possible.

▶ Stress tears you down.

▶ Recovery builds you up.

▶ Transformation is the result.

Skip recovery, and stress eats you alive. Your hormones spiral. Cortisol stays high. Belly fat sticks. Hunger spikes. Sleep collapses. Injuries creep in.

But when you recover right, everything flips:

▶ Muscles rebuild stronger.

▶ Fat burns instead of stores.

▶ Energy returns.

▶ Your brain clears.

▶ Your willpower strengthens.

Recovery isn't optional. It's the other half of the mission.

Nutrition – The Blueprint of Recovery

Here's where most people screw up: they treat nutrition like gas for the workout. Wrong.

Nutrition is the blueprint for what happens after the workout.

▶ Protein repairs muscle fibers and keeps metabolism high.

▶ Carbs restore glycogen so your muscles and brain function.

▶ Fats regulate hormones like testosterone and cortisol.

▶ Micronutrients (zinc, magnesium, vitamin D, potassium) are the spark plugs for healing.

▶ Hydration + electrolytes prevent cramping, dizziness, and the crashes most mistake for "weakness."

Every time I puked mid-run, it wasn't cardio's fault. It was my fault. My nutrition was sabotage.

When I fixed it, the war changed.

Stress vs Recovery – The Physiology

▶ Fight-or-flight mode (stress): Cortisol spikes, blood sugar floods, heart pounds, digestion shuts down. Great in a sprint. Terrible if you never escape it.

▶ Rest-and-digest mode (recovery): Cortisol drops, heart slows, blood flow shifts to repair, immunity kicks in.

If you live in fight-or-flight, you store fat, burn muscle, and shorten your fuse.

If you master recovery, you burn fat, grow muscle, and expand your capacity.

Healing Timeframes

You can't cheat biology. Every tissue heals on a clock:

▶ Muscles: 24–72 hours depending on intensity.

▶ Tendons/ligaments: slower, days to weeks.

▶ Skin/fascia: hydration, collagen, circulation dependent.

When I skipped recovery, my calves screamed every day. They never healed. But when I finally respected biology, gave them food, rest, and time the pain eased and progress skyrocketed.

Recovery Tools That Work

Here's what actually works (tested on myself, confirmed by science):

- Stretching & mobility: fascia health, joint freedom.
- Banana/fruit pre-run: fast carbs + potassium.
- Protein within 60 minutes: non-negotiable repair.
- Electrolytes during long sweats: salt, magnesium, potassium.
- Active recovery: light walking, cycling, yoga.
- Sleep: 7–9 hours. Growth hormone won't release without it.
- Mindset reset: journaling, meditation, breath work to calm cortisol.

The Boring Stuff Is the Real Hero

The highlight reels never show it.

Nobody posts pictures of the banana before the run.
Or the 10 minutes of stretching.
Or the glass of water before bed.
Or the protein shake when you don't feel like it.

But that's what wins the war.
Not the puke. Not the grind porn.
The boring stuff.

Your Recovery War Plan

Daily Checklist

- Sleep: 7–9 hours. Non-negotiable.
- Protein: 1–2g per pound of goal weight.

- ▶ Hydration: ½ oz per pound of bodyweight + electrolytes.
- ▶ Mobility: 10 minutes daily.
- ▶ Post-workout fuel: protein + carb.
- ▶ Mind reset: 5–10 minutes breath or gratitude.

Follow this, and your body doesn't just survive workouts, it transforms from them.

Lock It In

Recovery isn't laziness. Recovery is discipline.

The Florida runs taught me this: puking wasn't proof. It was punishment for ignoring recovery.

The proof came when I humbled myself to the boring, consistent, science-backed recovery that rebuilt me.

And when I locked it in, everything changed.

I stopped breaking down.

- ▶ I started building up.
- ▶ My body transformed.
- ▶ My mind stabilized.
- ▶ My mission advanced.

Because you don't win the war by grinding 24/7.

You win it by recovering like a professional.

The grind doesn't make you.

The recovery does.

From Spectator to Doer:

But Cristian Why does Watching Drain You?

I'll never forget this.

A client walked into one of my sessions fired up about an NFL game he had just watched. He broke down the plays like a pro analyst, the stats, the highlight reel, who fumbled, who scored. For fifteen straight minutes, it was like listening to a podcast.

An hour later, that same guy told me he felt exhausted. His energy was gone, his recovery was off, and he couldn't figure out why.

That's when it hit me.

He wasn't tired because he trained too hard. He was tired because he lived like a spectator, not a doer.

Spectators Burn Energy They Don't Even Use

Here's the science: watching sports or even scrolling highlight reels tricks your brain into feeling like you're participating.

When you watch athletes, your brain fires off mirror neurons, the same cells that activate when you actually perform the action. That means you burn mental energy, get a hit of dopamine, even feel the cortisol spikes... without moving a single muscle.

It's a chemical illusion. You feel like you "did something," but your body knows you didn't.

That's why so many people feel drained after binging TV, gaming, or scrolling. Your nervous system is firing like you just ran a marathon, but your body never got the payoff, no training, no growth, no recovery.

Spectating is spiritual junk food. It fills your head, but it starves your life.

163

The Doing Difference

Think about the athletes you watch:

▶ They don't just train; they recover like their paycheck depends on it.
▶ They fuel with precision.
▶ They sleep like it's part of the contract.
▶ They treat their body like a business.

Meanwhile, spectators eat chips, drink beer, and yell at the TV like that's effort.

If you want proof of what separates the two? It's recovery. The doers fuel, stretch, sleep, hydrate, breathe. The spectators just talk.

The secret is this: when you train, eat, and live like the people you admire, one day you stop watching. You start being.

Spectating Steals Your Recovery

Here's something most people never consider:
Spectating wrecks recovery.

Why? Because while you're on the couch watching another man's highlight reel, you're stealing time from your own recovery cycle.

▶ Late-night games = poor sleep quality → higher cortisol → slower repair.
▶ Game-day food = sabotage fuel (beer, wings, chips) → inflammation spikes → worse healing.
▶ Emotional stress of fandom = cortisol dump → cravings, fat storage, agitation.

So when my client told me he felt drained, I knew exactly why. He wasn't recovering from training, he was recovering from spectating.

The Psychology of Spectatorship

There's a deeper layer here.

People watch because it's easier than doing.

It's safer to admire someone else's courage than face the battlefield of your own life.

But here's the truth: no one remembers the guy who knew all the stats. No one builds legacy as a commentator on other men's greatness. Legacy comes from the man or woman who takes the field of their own life.

My Wake-Up Call

When I was 370 pounds, I used to spectate too. Sports, shows, scrolling. I watched other men win while I sat in silence losing my own battles.

I knew more about their stats than my own health. More about their schedules than my own meals. More about their plays than my own plan.

That's when it hit me: spectating was killing me.

I didn't need another highlight. I needed to become one.

From Couch to Creator

Here's the challenge I gave that client, and now I'm giving you:

1. Audit your hours. How much time do you spend watching other people live? Sports, shows, social media, log it.
2. Flip one block. If you watch three hours of football, flip one into training, meal prep, or recovery work. That's 52 extra hours a year added to your mission.
3. Consume like a pro. Athletes watch film to improve. If you're spectating, do it with intent. Study form, discipline, resilience then apply it.

4. Build your highlight reel. Every workout logged, every meal tracked, every recovery step taken, that's your film. Build a reel worth rewatching.

Lock It In

Here's the truth no spectator wants to hear:

▶ Talking about other people's wins doesn't change your life.
▶ Watching the highlight reel doesn't heal your body.
▶ Admiring someone else's proof doesn't build your own.

The transition from spectator to doer is where everything changes. And the bridge between the two is recovery.

Because when you start training, eating, and recovering like the people you watch, you stop watching altogether. You start being.

And the day you stop spectating and start doing? That's the day you go from tired to unstoppable. It's time and you know it. So get off that sideline stop watching and come play.

The Currency of Time

The Equalizer

Every person you've ever admired from Navy SEALs to billionaires to world-class athletes, wakes up with the exact same twenty-four hours you do. Not a second more, not a second less. That truth is both brutal and liberating. Brutal because there are no excuses. Liberating because no one has an advantage over you when it comes to time.

Money isn't equal. Some people are born into wealth. Connections aren't equal. Some people have family names that open doors before they even knock. Even genetics aren't equal. But time? Time is fair. You and I, the president and the janitor, the millionaire and the man drowning in debt, we all open our eyes each morning with the exact same deposit: 86,400 seconds.

And here's the secret: it resets every single day. No carryover, no rollover minutes, no do-overs. You don't lose yesterday's mistakes. You don't bank tomorrow's opportunities. You only have today.

My Wake-Up Call

When I was losing 200 pounds, time management became the battlefield where I either won or lost the day. People always ask, "How did you find the time to train, to eat clean, to rebuild your life?"

The truth is, I didn't find time. I made time.

Back then, I was working long hours, carrying debt, battling my health, and trying to be present for my family. There were days I wanted to believe the lie that I was just too busy, that the schedule was stacked against me. But then I had a wake-up call.

One morning, staring at myself in the mirror, exhausted from excuses, I realized:

No one was going to give me more time.
No one was going to extend my clock.
The twenty-four hours I had were the same as everyone else's.

And if someone else could train, eat, and build their dream with the same twenty-four, then so could I.

The Daily Reset

I want you to think about this: every single morning the scoreboard resets to zero.

- ▶ Yesterday's failures don't disqualify you.
- ▶ Yesterday's wins don't guarantee you anything today.

> ▶ The clock doesn't care if you're rich or broke, fit or overweight, motivated or depressed.

The day is new, and the seconds are fresh.

That's the ultimate mercy of time: it wipes the slate clean at midnight. But it's also the ultimate test: what will you do with it now?

The Lie of "Catching Up"

Have you ever told yourself, "I'm behind"? Behind in life, behind in money, behind in fitness, behind on your dreams? I've said it a thousand times. But here's the hard truth: you can't be behind on time. Nobody can.

Time isn't a race where someone else gets a head start. You're not losing hours to the guy across the street. He's not ahead. He just chose differently with his twenty-four than you did.

This truth changed me: I can't control yesterday. I can't control what's lost. But I can control the next minute, the next hour, the next choice. That's all that ever matters.

A Moment I'll Never Forget

Let me take you to a day that punched me in the gut.

I was standing in the hospital, waiting for results after a doctor told me I might not live to see forty if I didn't change. The walls felt cold. Time felt heavy. I remember staring at the clock on the wall, second hand ticking. And for the first time in my life, I didn't just see time as background noise, I saw it as currency I'd been wasting.

Every tick was a dollar leaving my account.
Every minute was a chance I'd never get back.
Every hour was a decision, invest it or burn it.

Right there, I made a promise: if I walked out of that hospital, I would never again say, "I don't have time." I'd stop pretending I was a victim of my schedule. I'd become the owner of my hours.

The System That Saved Me

Here's the system I lived by: Prioritize, Protect, and Produce.

1. Prioritize.

> Every morning, I wrote down the top three things that would move me forward. Not thirty. Not twenty. Three. If I finished those three, the day was a win.

2. Protect.

> I guarded my calendar like it was my life because it was. I turned off notifications. I said no to distractions. I cut out anything that stole hours without paying me back.

3. Produce.

> Then I executed. Not perfect. Not always motivated. But consistent. One meal prepped. One workout logged. One page written. One call made.

This rhythm, repeated daily, is how I lost 200 pounds, built a business, and rebuilt my life.

The Weight of Excuses

I meet men all the time who tell me, "I just don't have the time."

I ask them: "How many hours did you spend scrolling your phone yesterday?"

"How many hours did you spend watching Netflix?"

"How many hours did you give to gossip, negativity, or worrying about things you can't control?"

The room goes silent.

The truth is, it's not about time. It's about choices. Every yes is a no to something else. Every wasted hour is an investment you'll never get back.

The Father's Lesson

One of the most influential lessons I learned about time came from my dad. He used to tell me, "Cristian, you can make money back. You can rebuild your health. You can even repair broken relationships. But you will never get back a lost hour."

I didn't listen back then. I thought time was endless. But standing at nearly 400 pounds, with a doctor telling me my time might be running out, I finally understood.

Time is the only non-renewable resource you'll ever have.

Practical Framework: The Daily Reset Rule

Here's a rule I want you to burn into your brain:

"Every day is a reset. Every day is a test. Every day is a choice."

- ▶ Reset: You start fresh. No excuses, no baggage.
- ▶ Test: The clock asks you, "What will you do today?"
- ▶ Choice: You decide what gets your energy and what doesn't.

If you want transformation in your body, your money, your marriage, your faith, it starts with owning your twenty-four. Nobody else can do it for you. Nobody else can steal your hours unless you hand them away.

When you stop saying "I don't have time" and start saying "This isn't a priority," your whole life changes. Because the truth is, you do have the time. You've always had the time. You just need to decide what matters enough to fill your hours.

The reset starts today. The clock is ticking. The only question is: what will you do with your twenty-four? Will you invest your own currency into building your life, or waste it spectating how others spend theirs?

Transformation?

When people think about transformation, they obsess over willpower. They believe the answer is pure grit, forcing themselves to make the right choice, white-knuckling through cravings, and powering through distractions.

But here's the truth most people miss: your environment is silently shaping 90% of your decisions before willpower even enters the room.

I didn't lose 200 pounds just because I became "stronger." I lost it because I redesigned the world around me so the right choices were easier, and the wrong choices were harder.

The Weight of a Kitchen

When I was nearly 400 pounds, my kitchen told the story of my struggle. Soda cans in the fridge. Chips in the pantry. Drive-thru bags on the counter. Every time I walked into that room, temptation whispered my name.

And here's the thing, to this day, I still face obstacles. But now I live by a rule: plan and stay proactive.

If I'm traveling, I decide beforehand what I'm eating. I don't "settle" for fast food, I'll run into Walmart, grab a rotisserie chicken, Greek yogurt, maybe some fruit, and that becomes my fallback plan.

It doesn't matter what field you're on or whose playground you're standing in, you own it. You take control. You choose the narrative.

Here's what most people don't realize: you don't have to fight temptation all day. You can remove it.

One of the first changes I made was clearing the junk out of my kitchen. No more sodas. No more chips. If I wanted junk food, I had to get in my car, drive across town, and buy it. Suddenly, "willpower" became easier because I designed my environment to support me instead of sabotage me.

The Circle Around You

It's not just about the kitchen. It's also about the people at your table.

Some of you are trying to transform your life while sitting at a table where every conversation is negative, every joke is self-destructive, every plan is small-minded. That environment is poisoning you slowly.

I had to learn the hard way that sometimes transformation means letting go of relationships that keep you stuck. Not because you hate those people, but because your future can't survive in the soil of your past.

When I surrounded myself with people who demanded more of me, who didn't let me play the victim, who called me higher, everything shifted. I rose to the level of my environment.

Environments Don't Lie

Here's something you need to burn into your brain: your environment always tells the truth about your priorities.

Look at your car. Is it trashed or clean? That says something about your habits.

Look at your bedroom. Is it chaos or order? That says something about your mindset.

Look at your calendar. Is it full of distractions or full of purpose? That says something about your direction.

We lie to ourselves with words all the time: "I'm disciplined. I'm focused. I'm serious." But our environment exposes the truth.

Design Your World for Momentum

Here's the good news: you don't have to rely on motivation if you design your environment to pull you forward.

- ▶ Want to read more? Put books where your phone usually sits.
- ▶ Want to train more? Put your workout clothes by your bed the night before.
- ▶ Want to eat better? Meal prep once so your fridge tells you "yes" instead of "no."

Success isn't about being the strongest fighter every day. It's about setting up the battlefield so you don't have to fight as hard.

The Hidden Environments

Most people think "environment" is just physical, your house, your office, your gym. But there are two more environments that matter just as much:

1. Digital Environment

> What voices fill your feed? Who are you following? Every scroll is shaping your belief system. If your feed is full of gossip, outrage, and distractions, don't be surprised when your mind feels cluttered and weak.

2. Mental Environment

> What stories are you rehearsing in your head every day? Are you replaying failures, insults, and fears? Or are you rehearsing

gratitude, vision, and possibilities? The environment in your head can be more toxic than any pantry.

The Law of Proximity

There's an old saying: "Show me your friends and I'll show you your future."

I'd take it further: "Show me your environment and I'll show you your destiny."

▶ If you spend your nights in bars, don't be shocked when your life revolves around alcohol.

▶ If you spend your hours around men who have no discipline, don't be shocked when you fall back into excuses.

▶ If you spend your energy in places that drain you, don't be shocked when you have nothing left for what matters.

But here's the flip side:

▶ Spend your time in the gym, and discipline starts to feel normal.

▶ Spend your time with visionaries, and dreaming bigger starts to feel possible.

▶ Spend your time in environments that demand growth, and growth becomes inevitable.

Final Word

Transformation isn't just about who you are. It's about where you are.

If you want to change your life, don't just rewrite your habits, redesign your environment. Create a kitchen that fuels your health, a calendar that reflects your purpose, a circle of people who pull you higher.

Because at the end of the day, you don't rise to the level of your intentions.

You fall to the level of your environment.

And if you want to win with your twenty-four hours, you'd better make sure the place you spend them is built to push you forward.

CONNECT WITH THE AUTHOR

Cristian Lopez is a veteran, best-selling author, and transformation expert who naturally lost 200 pounds in one year. After overcoming addiction, a life-threatening diagnosis, and financial struggles, Cristian rebuilt his life with discipline, structure, and a relentless no-excuses approach.

Today, known worldwide as The Traction Coach, Cristian equips men and veterans to break through excuses, build unstoppable momentum, and take control of their health, wealth, and future. His coaching, bootcamps, and speaking events are built on the same principles that transformed his own life.

Cristian's mission is simple: to prove that lasting transformation is possible for anyone willing to commit.

Start your own transformation and access Cristian's newest book offer at TractionC.com

Stay connected: Email Cristian directly at Cristian@Aivex.ai